God's Prescription for Mental Health and Religion

Smile if You Truly Believe Your Religion

E. Rae Harcum

Hamilton Books
A member of
The Rowman & Littlefield Publishing Group
Lanham · Boulder · New York · Toronto · Plymouth, UK

Hamilton Books
4501 Forbes Boulevard
Suite 200
Lanham, Maryland 20706
Hamilton Books Acquisitions Department (301) 459-3366

Estover Road
Plymouth PL6 7PY
United Kingdom

Printed in the United States of America
British Library Cataloging in Publication Information Available

Library of Congress Control Number: 2010929917
ISBN: 978-0-7618-5201-8 (paperback : alk. paper)
eISBN: 978-0-7618-5202-5

Dedication

This book is lovingly dedicated to the late Rosalyn Moore Hahn, my wife's cousin and a dear friend of the family. Rosalyn taught Sunday school continuously for over 55 years. She worked tirelessly as a volunteer all of her life in more venues than I can name. In 1994, she was named volunteer of the year for the Commonwealth of Virginia. Her life was truly characterized by loving service to others. We miss her as a dear friend and relative and as an always-dependable helper.

Contents

Preface

A respected social worker once said to me about a mutual friend, "If she would just start thinking about others, instead of herself all of the time, she would not have so many physical and psychological problems." Indeed, this one brief proposition summarizes the central lesson of this book: God's prescription, the highway to mental health of individuals and of society is the high way—God's way—which includes selfless devotion and service to others. To be sure, rigorous psychological research shows that people who believe, as we do, in a loving and supportive God do in fact enjoy better mental health. Thus, this book shows how good mental health is so closely tied to good spiritual health.

The main thrust of the book is to urge the reader to focus on the message, not just to think and *be* good, but to *do* good for others. To be sure, a Christian should be good, but, as I read Jesus' keynote passage, He emphasized good behavior as necessary for triumphant living.

This powerful message is conveyed also in the second keynote passage from Rollo May, a noted author in psychological science. May says that we find the good life that we do not seek for ourselves specifically and exactly because we have not misdirected our lives toward seeking personal rewards. I call this fundamental truth of life, from the Bible and from experts in psychology, the "Paradox of Christian Living."

Thus, the present book is both a religious work and a summary of some basic psychological truths for joyous living. Such a claim for a joint religious and psychological enterprise will probably not surprise religious authors, but it will probably astonish the traditional authors of psychological science. Historically, the religious authors have opened wide the door to psychological science, whereas the authors of psychology traditionally have closed the door of their science to religion because they consider it to be a non-rigorous distraction.

As a psychologist, I wish to help change the general thinking of the profession in this respect. Indeed, the change has already begun, as recent publications show. I argue, of course, that the basic ideas of psychological science and religion must surely be mutually supportive because the science of psychology also comes from God. Both are fully committed to truth. Thus, this book advocates the use of power from the Holy Bible, verified and reinforced by principles from rigorous science, for guidance in our stressful world at the beginning of the 21st century.

We know that the Holy Bible surely guides us to future eternal happiness in Heaven. The present thesis is that it also provides inexhaustible guidance for mental health and happiness in our lives on earth, right here and right now. As Rev. George Insley, Jr., a retired pastor of the United Methodist Church, said in a sermon on June 29, 2003, at Tabernacle Church in Poquoson, Virginia: "If you truly believe your religion, smile." So, believe it; the Christian message is an entirely positive view of the world.

The healing guidelines in the Bible—both psychological and theological—flow from the core mandates of the Great Commandment to love God and to love our neighbors as ourselves. And love necessarily implies service to others. To be sure, love is actually validated through service. With true love there is no need to keep score as to who has benefited most from a personal connection of service. Everyone is the better for it.

Undoubtedly, those Christians who commit themselves fully to the combined power of the Scriptures and psychological science can expect more peace and joy in life. So, you can put yourself on the highway to mental health and happiness on earth, as a sure side effect of your commitment to love and to serve. But, if your true goals of life are selfish, you destroy God's prescription for your highway to health, which He, out of His infinite love, has given to you.

Acknowledgments

This book owes special debts to many dedicated servants of God. Particularly, my good friend, Vince Sutlive, a Methodist Minister and former missionary, has been a never-ending source of knowledge, wisdom and inspiration. Barbara Freeman and Gwen Perkins, both informed and committed Christians, read early drafts and offered extremely helpful suggestions. As always, my thinking has been guided by the thoughtful comments of my wife, Phoebe. Other debts are too numerous to be mentioned here. Nevertheless, I remain fully responsible for the contents of this book.

I thank the International Bible Society and Zondervan Publishing House for permission to quote from the New International Version of the Bible. All Biblical quotations are from this source.

Plan of the Book

The first chapter of this book emphasizes that God made all things, including the science of psychology. Thus, the science of psychology and religious faith join together in seeking truth and the improvement of life on earth—i.e., mental health. Chapter 2 argues that some psychological theories on the nature of man are incompatible with Judeo-Christian religion, but one theory, called Humanism, is consistent with that religion.

Chapter 3 calls for Christian thinking in the conduct of our lives on Earth. Chapter 4 suggests ways for Christians to become better Christians. Chapter 5 continues to suggest how a person can become a better Christian. Chapter 6 emphasizes the importance of forgiveness as a condition of mental health. Chapter 7 stresses the importance of personal choice in selecting Christian responses. Chapter 8 describes how the nature of our human brain is related to the development of morality and virtue. Chapter 9 discusses ways in which Christian behavior can improve our quality of life. Chapter 10 asserts that a life of loving will lead to a preponderance of feelings of happiness and well-being in life.

The book is summarized in the Final Words, which say that love leads to virtue, a healthy conscience, a positive outlook on life and confidence in the future.

Keynote Messages

Then Jesus said to his disciples, "If anyone would come after me, he must deny himself and take up his cross and follow me. For whoever wants to save his life will lose it, but whoever loses his life for me will find it." (Matthew 16: 24-25)

Therapy should enable the patient to rediscover himself, or discover himself on a level where he can choose values that commit himself to something in life, a level where he can love or at least know when he is not loving, and where he can experience some gratification. (Rollo May, p. 26, in M. H. Hall, September, 1967, An interview with Mr. Humanist, Rollo May. *Psychology Today, 1*, 24-29, 72-73.)

PART I. GOD'S LAWS

Chapter 1

In The Beginning

I begin this book with the classic story of the old man whose home was seriously threatened by rapidly rising floodwaters. The old man, despite desperate entreaties by his friends, refused to leave his home. He trusted absolutely that his God would save him. The old gentleman was sitting on his front porch, watching the waters rise, when a neighbor in a jeep stopped in front of his house and offered him a ride to safe ground. The old man declined, saying that the Lord would keep him safe. After the water had risen yet higher, another friend rowed by in a boat, and offered to ferry him to safety. From his second-story window, the old fellow refused, again asserting that God would take care of him. Then, the flood increased to the point that the old one had to take refuge on his roof. As the water now lapped about his heels, a helicopter came to hover over him, and the pilot begged him to climb aboard, because additional flooding was anticipated. Still, the old man refused, vowing that he would eternally trust in the Lord to keep him from harm. Finally, the flood washed over the house, and the old man drowned.

Because he had displayed so much faith and trust in the Lord, naturally the drowned man went to heaven. As soon as he arrived, he rushed straight to God, and complained that he had maintained his absolute trust to the end, but God had failed to rescue him. Then, God said sadly, "My son, you are mistaken. Out of my deep love and compassion for you, on three separate occasions I sent vehicles for your rescue. I sent first a jeep, then a boat and finally I sent a helicopter. But, on each occasion you firmly declined my help."

The lesson of the story is powerful: Surely, God can move in mysterious ways, but sometimes His ways seem not at all extraordinary. Indeed, on occasion, they can appear to be downright ordinary to us. So, God is still the Creator of all things, of even those things that do not seem miraculous.

As the Bible says in Genesis, God gave human beings the capacity to understand and to act, so that we might have dominion over His creations on earth. God was not sparing. His gifts to us include both rational and intuitive, scientific and religious avenues for understanding and saving our world. In sum, both the unfamiliar and the pedestrian come from God.

Perhaps the old man in the story was actually arrogant in presupposing how God was going to save him, or even that saving his life was part of God's plan.

In any case, it hardly seems Christian to demand of God that we control His plans, that we will accept and acknowledge only outright miracles that obviously must come from Him. We must remember that both the seeming miracles and the commonplaces of science come from Him.

The present book maintains that the field of science—which we claim to understand—and the field of religion—which we do not claim to understand—

are both fully legitimate under God. Neither can be reduced to the other. As a consequence, this book is not about the psychology *of* religion, but about psychology *and* religion. It is about the joint, integrated use of psychology and theology to achieve a virtuous, happy life.

A virtuous life is a happy life because the Word of God is also a blueprint for psychological health and wholeness. Think about it! This blueprint is a limitless source of power for helping others, and thus also for power to help oneself, as well. In addition to the taproot of the Great Commandment, there are many specific Biblical principles for the psychological guidance of human behavior. For example, the keynote quotation from Matthew provides the most important idea for promoting mental health on earth: Focus your attention on love and selfless service to others, and not on personal wishes, pleasures and privileges. Thus, the improvement of both self and society begins indirectly with the desire to become more outwardly directed in thinking about the welfare of God's people. In fact, personal mental health is a beautiful side effect—a natural fall-out of a Christian life. This happy conclusion is supported by the results of psychological research, as will be discussed later in this book.

Indeed, the importance of actually doing God's word was recently emphasized by Willard, who argued that obedience to Jesus' teachings was essential for well-being in our world today, as follows:

> More than any other single thing, in any case, *the practical irrelevance of actual obedience to Christ* accounts for the weakened effect of Christianity in the world today, with its increasing tendency to emphasize political and social action as the primary way to serve God. It also accounts for the practical irrelevance of Christian faith to individual character development and overall personal sanity and well-being.[1]

This idea of doing versus simply believing was supported by Henderson and Casper. In their book, the Christian pastor, Jim, after visiting churches across the country, discusses religion and evaluates each religious service with Casper, an Atheist. After their visit to the church of Mark Driscoll, a fast-growing, "emerging" church in Seattle, Casper observes:

> What I'm trying to say is I'm hearing a promise of personal happiness through a series of things *not* to do rather than things to do. I guess you'd say it's a call *not to act*, rather than to act. Driscoll's pitch seems to be that to be happy and achieve heaven, just say no to sin. Is that in tune with what Jesus said? . . .
> I understand that Christians believe that Jesus was free of sin, but my impression is that he didn't focus on that. He wasn't like, 'Look at me! No sin at all! Be just like me!' Based on what I've read, his main thing was going out and helping the poor in spirit and those who were suffering, and instructing others to do the same.

Yes, I think I could picture Jesus high-five-ing you on that one.[2]

The personal benefit of giving religion away to others is greater if the insight of others is gained primarily from personal effort. To be sure, every enduring faith must be individually crafted. No one on earth—no teacher, no preacher, no author—can give anyone a packaged religious faith that truly matters. We authors can only help you with your own search for personal meaning. I pray that my witness and arguments may help you to establish beliefs that will bring you personal salvation, and also the psychological peace on earth that goes naturally with it.

I feel that I write with some inspiration as a committed Christian. I do not believe that my faith is unique. I have been a Christian and a member of the United Methodist Church for over 70 years. Therefore, I offer a witness to a personal faith, bolstered by the wise counsel and spiritual examples of many far more knowledgeable pastors, teachers and friends. For example, the inspiration, knowledge and encouragement of my good friend, Vince Sutlive, of the anthropology department at the College of William and Mary, also a Methodist minister and former missionary, have been invaluable to me in times of personal trial. That is what faith and friends do for you in times of trial.

I also claim the credentials of a general psychologist, with an extensive background in research and in teaching scientific methodology. After training as a Ph.D. in psychology, I worked as a psychologist for over 38 years. For years, I was satisfied to keep my two domains of experience and belief essentially separate, as parallel approaches to two different kinds of knowledge. In later years, however, I became dissatisfied with that thinking, and have tried to bring the two categories of experience—the nominally scientific and the nominally religious—together in my thinking and writing. This means to infuse religion-compatible thinking into my writing in psychology, as well as the present effort to infuse psychological thought into a basically religious book.

Such an effort toward intellectual and spiritual integration reflects a growing national trend among psychologists. Rebecca Clay, writing for the *A.P. A. Monitor* of the American Psychological Association, described how psychologists historically tended to distrust religion, blaming it for all kinds of problems in mental health.[3] Clay reported that only about one-third of psychologists claimed to orient their lives around their religious beliefs, in contrast to about three-fourths of the general population.[4] But Clay also reported new evidence that this traditional negative view by psychologists toward religion has begun to change in a positive direction.[5] A stream of new books on the value of spirituality in mental health and psychotherapy supports this conclusion.[6]

Applied Science vs. Miracles

In this section, I argue that God has ordained scientific laws so that we can use applied science to improve ourselves and the world around us. There is nothing basically wrong with praying for miracles, of course. But, miracles are not the only way that God can produce change in the world or in persons. He can inspire us to use our rational and emotional abilities to adapt scientific principles for instituting valued change.

The very existence of miracles does prove God's occasional willingness to suspend His physical laws. Because God's miracles, by definition, violate His ordained physical laws, I infer that He is not likely to dispense them easily for the instant gratification of each Christian upon request. Indeed, a miracle that benefits one Christian may inconvenience, or even harm, his or her neighbor. To take a trivial example, God cannot be pleased when one Christian prays for a miracle that would enable one football team to defeat the team supported by another Christian. I presume that God would prefer that we use the earthly resources that He has already made available to us for winning football games through our own resources.

Undoubtedly, our world must be controlled by impersonal physical laws. When God ordained those laws, He did not make them conditional upon the desires of individual Christians. Christians cannot expect to isolate or insulate themselves from the ordered world of God. To be sure, discord and tragedies disrupt personal peace and joy from time to time. In fact, Christians ought to have their peace and joy disturbed by the inevitable misfortunes and sufferings of fellow travelers on this earth, particularly those misfortunes that we can mitigate or eliminate by our own efforts.

Some years ago, the psychologist George Miller used the phrase "giving psychology away" to refer to the process of educating the public in the use of psychology to improve our society.[7] He argued that we should not simply follow without direction or plan certain procedures for dealing with people. Rather, we should deliberately design, or re-design, those procedures in order to make a better world. He argued that the principles of psychology will not be effective unless they are thoroughly understood by those who would apply them for practical use.

The same is true for the application of Christianity. Miller's ideas are entirely consistent with our goal to give Christianity away. Evangelism is our great commission and priority. We must be evangelists with the best understanding, sophistication and dedication in religion, as well as in psychology, that we can muster.

The present book combines the nominally religious and the nominally psychological perspectives in understanding the relationships among people. Although the two perspectives are different in some respects, the ultimate goals are to improve the relationships among the peoples of the earth. While the science of psychology cannot discover relationships that are contrary to, or outside of, God's laws, it does provide different methods for studying human behavior and different terminologies and conceptualizations of the relationships.

Increased understanding of God's human creation, by whatever means God has made available to us, develops our personal power for living a Christian life of service to others. Although the word "power" has come today to have bad connotations in the context of relationships among people, we should not think of it in such a way. The word generally refers to the ability to act, the capability of producing an effect. So, the empowered person has the ability to overcome various sources of resistance in order to accomplish the work of the Lord.

The ability to harness Christian power is itself power. The Christian must be able to make good decisions when there are many alternative paths for choice, some of which are Christian, but others are not. Therefore, Christian power is not just about strength and energy, but also about cognitive awareness and reasoned judgment. In other words, we must be smart in our use of the power that we control. We must look ahead at the likely outcomes. We must know how to implement our beliefs in the homes, in the schools and in the work places and marketplaces of the world. The supplementary study of psychological science will help us in that vital task.

Religion and Mental Health

God made all things in Heaven and on earth. Therefore, He established all of the laws—spiritual, mental, physical—by which this universe operates. Consequently, a second, rather redundant, assertion is that God made possible the science of psychology, and thus human promotion of mental health on earth. God wants us to be happy, as He has taught us how to be happy. Using the skills and tools that He has provided, psychologists try to discover God's laws of human mental activity and behavior in order to reduce human suffering, and to gain true happiness for all.

Many of God's laws are explicitly stated in the Bible. For example, the keynote quotation from Matthew, describing what I call "the Paradox of Christian Living," anticipates the conclusion of the famous psychologist, Rollo May, also quoted in a keynote message.[8] The successful human being has been able to commit himself or herself to something important in life, and to know love. It is critical that the thing of value is outside and beyond individual personal pleasure. May was not referring specifically to religion, but generally to focusing one's thoughts and energy toward something other than one's own personal welfare, and to a focus on learning to love. To be sure, for the committed Christian, religion does exactly those things.

These parallels between religious and psychological well-being must be emphasized, because the anti-religious writers in psychology have been much more successful in getting their opposite, negative and destructive, messages before the public. Unfortunately, many Christians have come to view all of the philosophical orientations in psychology as steps toward science and secularism, and therefore away from spirituality. For example, the psychological view that emphasizes the unique human nature of mankind—i.e., the one called Humanism —is seen by some religionists as a step away from religion, rather than as a potential step toward it. They forget that Christ was also human. Human beings are constructed to be a little less than the angels. We are not machines or robots; in particular, we have the ability to make personal choices. Therefore, increased understanding of human nature does not remove or replace the need or the possibility of God. The celebration of our humanity is sinful only when it attempts to give mankind the final authority and power in the universe.

To be sure, the theoretical views of some psychologists—the Behaviorists[9] and the Psychoanalysts[10]—are incompatible with Judeo-Christian thinking. But the views of other psychologists, the Humanists[11] surely are compatible with a religious life. Therefore, the opposition to religion of some psychologists does not mean that the whole field of psychology itself must be anti-religious.

To say that the Humanistic view of psychologists is compatible with religion is not to say that it is religious, however. This book urges the Humanists in psychology to take another step upward, to holiness, to a life in the Judeo-Christian tradition.

Recently, there has been an increased interest by psychologists in the empirical determination of the effects of religious beliefs and practices on mental health. Surprisingly, the actual functional relationship has not been easy to discover. A number of complex procedural and definitional problems have prevented an easy answer to the question.

One problem in establishing the true relationship is the difficulty of actually specifying such things as the religious beliefs themselves, not to say the nature of mental health. For example, mental health may be defined by some scholars simply as not having a need for religion, as just being liberal in attitude and maintaining an open mind. Or, perhaps paradoxically, some may even champion the idea that mental health involves a failure to hold to strong beliefs of any sort. In such cases, the sheer definition of the terms completely determines the empirical relationship between religious beliefs and mental health. Therefore, the answer from such mental activity is not relevant to our question.

A second problem in assessing the relationship between religion and mental health is that persons with problems in their lives may turn to religion to secure help with those very problems. In such a case, the relationship would have to be inverse, because the overt practice of religion was initially caused by the absence of mental health. The empirical research could reveal the residual presence of the lingering problems, even though the religious beliefs and practices may truly have been effective in helping to deal with or alleviate those original problems.

A third obstacle is that the answer to the relation between religion and mental health may depend upon the particular kind of religious orientation that is involved. Some religious beliefs and practices may support mental health, and some may not.

Despite the research problems, a general positive relationship has been concluded. For example, Oman and Thoresen reached the following conclusion about the relationship between the practice of religion and health: "An important development in the scientific study of religion over the past decade has been an increasing number of studies that have persuasively documented positive relationships between religious involvement and physical and mental health outcomes . . . ."[12]

Mahoney and Tarakeshwar conclude from their analysis of empirical results relating religion to marriage and family life that, "In conclusion, available empirical research indicates that greater religiousness is linked to more positive marital and family functioning."[13] It should be kept in mind that this conclusion refers to religion in general, and not to a specific form or practice of religion.

Miller and Kelley also emphasize the positive effects of religion on mental health.[14] Nevertheless, they point out the complexity of the empirical relationships and the question of whether a relationship proves that mental health is a cause or an effect of mental health. Indeed, Hartz reminds us that an empirical positive statistical correlation between the practice of religion and measures of mental and physical health does not prove that there is an actual causal relationship of one on the other.[15] Other evidence is necessary.

The value of religion for mental health is strongly implied by the assertions of many psychotherapists who attest to the value of religion in psychotherapy.[16] The causal inference comes directly from their clinical experiences. As Hart emphatically asserts,

> Sound spirituality is itself therapeutic, and from its commitment to fullness of life it supports every therapeutic effort. At the same time, psychology harbors insights and instruments useful in the attainment of spirituality's goals. These two human endeavors have the resources both to enrich and to critique each other in helpful ways.[17]

Thus, he says of psychology and spirituality, "Both seek to liberate people from what shackles them, and lead them toward a more fulfilling life."[18]

Other psychotherapists agree. For example, as Safranske concludes: "Advances in clinical practice, drawing on the scholarship within the psychology of religion, offer the possibility of addressing and incorporating religious and spiritual dimension, which are salient in the lives of most individuals, into clinical practice, and encourages (sic) a more comprehensive approach to human suffering and healing."[19]

Finally, Kahle and Robbins concluded from their clinical practice that: "Many of our clients have reported they have made gains with spiritually inclusive therapy that they never made with more traditionally therapeutic approaches."[20]

There is also evidence of a mixed sort. For example, Hart argues that religion can be harmful as well as helpful, as follows:

> Religion is a dangerous thing. It can do great harm, as well as great good. What makes it dangerous is its immense power, which derives

> from its appeal to the Absolute or Ultimate as source for what it says and does. Religion signs God's name to what it proclaims, and therefore demands total allegiance. What it fails to acknowledge is that it is often mere human ideas to which it assigns God's authority.[21]

In addition to social evils, such as religious wars, persecution and abuses of power, Hart points out that, on an "individual level, it is not hard to find persons whose religious beliefs are doing them more harm than good, causing more blockage and pain than freedom, joy, or peace."[22]

These facts suggest that the effects of religion may depend upon the very type of religion that is involved. In fact, the answer to that very question is actually the empirical cornerstone of the present book: Only a religion based on the necessary centrality of love is positively related to good mental health.[23] *Those persons who believe in a personal, loving God, who cares for His people and can be depended upon, do in fact have happier, less troubled lives*. Such good religion does not view God as a purveyor of restrictive rules of conduct, but as a Shepherd who desires and promotes the welfare of His flock. Jesus made this truth very clear, as follows:

> Therefore Jesus said again, 'I tell you the truth, I am the gate for the sheep. All who ever came before me were thieves and robbers, but the sheep did not listen to them. I am the gate; whoever enters through me will be saved. He will come in and go out, and find pasture. The thief comes only to steal and kill and destroy; I have come that they may have life, and have it to the full.
> 'I am the good Shepherd. The good shepherd lays down his life for the sheep.'[24]

Conclusion

Indeed, the above considerations underscore the reasons that a causal relation between the practice of religion and the manifestation of mental health has been difficult to prove. For example, the study of Ventis showed a positive relationship between mental health and "good religion."[25] Presumably, good religion includes the practice of sacrificial service to others. Hart firmly supports this conclusion. He describes the advocation of Christian service by St. Ignatius Loyola, the founder of the Jesuit order of the Roman Catholic Church, as follows:

> He thought the greatest worship we could offer God was to put ourselves at the service of others, and that we could do that in the midst of the world without losing our prayerful contact with God because God was in the world, permeating all things. He thought that the best context for spiritual growth was not in a silent and sequestered space, but in the performance of Christian service, in interaction with others,

> for there we would be challenged to develop all the virtues.[26]

Therefore, this "good religion" contributes to all good things, including good mental health. Good religion involves a commitment to these particular convictions about our God, and a love and loyalty to the God of those convictions. The present book engages in a war of ideas against those psychologists who oppose what I have called good religion. The Christian convictions do open the gates to happiness on earth, as well as to the joys of Heaven.

Notes

1. Dallas Willard, *The Divine Conspiracy: Rediscovering Our Hidden Life in God* (New York: Harper San Francisco, 1998), xv.
2. Jim Henderson and Matt Cooper, *Jim and Casper go to Church: Frank Conversations about Faith, Churches, and Well-Meaning Christians* (Carol Stream, IL: Barna Books, 2007), 100.
3. Rebecca A. Clay, Psychologists' faith in religion begins to grow. *A.P.A. Monitor 27* (8) (1996a), 1, 48. Rebecca A. Clay, Religion and psychology share ideals and beliefs. *A.P.A. Monitor,* 27, 8 (1996b), 47.
4. Clay, Religion and psychology share ideals and beliefs.
5. Clay, Psychologists' faith in religion begins to grow.
6. Gary W. Hartz, *Spirituality and Mental Health: Clinical Applications* (Binghamton, NY: The Haworth Press, 2009). P. Kahle and J. M. Robbins, *The Power of Spirituality in Therapy: Integrating Spiritual and Religious Beliefs in Mental Health Practice* (Binghamton, NY: The Haworth Press, 2004). *Handbook of the Psychology of Religion and Spirituality*, eds. Raymond F. Paloutzian and Crystal L. Park (New York: The Guilford Press, 2005). Edward P. Safranske, The Psychology of Religion in Clinical and Counseling Psychology. In *Handbook of the Psychology of Religion and Spirituality,* eds. Raymond F. Paloutzian and Crystal Park (New York: The Guilford Press, 2005), 496-514.
7. George Miller, Psychology as a means of monitoring human welfare. *American Psychologist,* 46, (1969), 1063-1075.
8. Holy Bible, New International Version (Grand Rapids: Zondervan Publishing House, 1973), Matthew 16: 24-25. M. H. Hall, An interview with "Mr. Humanist," Rollo May, *Psychology Today*, 1, (1967), 24-29, 72-73.
9. John B. Watson, Psychology as the Behaviorist views it. *Psychological Review*, 20 (1913), 158-177.
10. Sigmund Freud, An *Outline of Psychoanalysis*, trans. J. Strachey (New York: Norton, 1949).
11. Carl R. Rogers, A theory of therapy, personality, and interpersonal relationships, as developed in the client-centered framework. In *Psychology: A Study of a Science*, Vol. 3, ed. S. Koch (New York: McGraw-Hill, 1959), 184-256.
12. Doug Oman and Carl Thoresen, Do religion and spirituality influence health? In *Handbook of the Psychology of Religion and Spirituality,* eds. Raymond F. Paloutzian and Crystal L. Park (New York: The Guilford Press, 2005), 435.
13. Annette Mahoney and Nalini Tarakeshwar, Religious role in marriage and parenting in daily life and during family crises. In *Handbook of the Psychology of Religion and Spirituality,* eds. Raymond F. Paloutzian and Crystal

L. Park (New York, The Guilford Press, 2005), 177-195, 191.

14. Lisa Miller and Brian S. Kelley, Relationship of Religiosity and Spirituality with Mental Health and Psychotherapy. In *Handbook of the Psychology of Religion and Spirituality,* eds. Raymond F. Paloutzian and Crystal L. Park (New York: The Guilford Press, 2005), 460-478.
15. Hartz, Spirituality and Mental Health.
16. Thomas Hart, *Hidden Spring: The Spiritual Dimension of Therapy* (2nd Ed.) (Minneapolis: Fortress Press, 2002). G. Miller, *Incorporating Spirituality into Counseling and Psychotherapy* (New York: Wiley, 2003). *Handbook of the Psychology of Religion and Spirituality* eds. Raymond F. Paloutzian and Crystal L. Park (New York: The Guilford Press, 2005). L. Sperry, *Spirituality in Clinical Practice: Incorporating the Spiritual Dimension in Psychotherapy and Counseling* (New York: Brunner, 2001).
17. Hart, *Hidden Spring*, 1.
18. *ibid*, 20
19. Safranske, The Psychology of Religion in Clinical and Counseling Psychology.
20. Kahle and Robbins, *The Power of Spirituality in Therapy*.
21. Hart, *Hidden Spring*, 29-30.
22. *ibid*, 30.
23. Clay, Psychologists' faith; Clay, Religion and Psychology.
24. Holy Bible, John 10: 7-11.
25. W. Laurance Ventis, The Relationship Between Religion and Mental Health. *Journal of Social Issues,* 5 (2), (1992), 33-48.
26. Hart, *HiddenSpring*, 18.

Chapter 2

Humanism and the Christian Model

Many Christians oppose the scientific views of psychology precisely because the science is not Christian. Indeed, scientific views are not Christian, nor should they be. That is to say, psychological theories should not be a substitute for religion.

There are three major psychological theories for describing the nature of human beings: Behaviorism,[1] Psychoanalysis,[2] and Humanism.[3] The Behavioristic view is divided into two subcategories: Strict Behaviorism[4] and Cognitive Behaviorism[5]. Among all of these theories, only the Humanistic view of people is fully compatible with religion.

These various theories are distinguished by many factors, such as the language to describe their concepts, but by only two major tenets. The first of these distinguishing ideas is the type of data that the theory will accept for validating their concepts. The Strict Behaviorists accept only so-called third-person data, meaning public events which can be observed and reported by anyone who is present.[6] The Cognitive Behaviorists, Psychoanalysts and Humanists also accept what is called second-person data, which are attempts to report personal experience.[7] These data are often referred to as the results of introspection. Finally, the approaches of Psychoanalysis and Humanism permit the use of so-called first-person data, which are personal experiences that really cannot be adequately described to another person. Thus, they are data that are available to only the one person who has actually had the experience.

Of course, the third-person data, acceptable to everyone, are most useful to science because such data are most objective. The first-person data are least useful scientifically because of the restricted subjective availability. But, these data may be more convincing to the one person who experienced them.

The second major difference among psychological theories is their position on the issue of free will vs. determinism. The principle of determinism says that behavior is caused entirely by the joint effects of heredity and environment. Thus, it denies freedom of will, meaning that the individual person cannot voluntarily choose to make a response other than the precise one produced by an interaction between his or her personal heredity and the existing personal environment. In contrast, the principle of free will says that a person can voluntarily exert an effect on his or her responses such that the response is *not entirely* controlled by his or her heredity and environment. That is, the person has a measure of freedom that will allow him or her to modify his or her responses voluntarily, to be partially or even wholly independent of external circumstances.

Only the Humanistic view in psychology accepts the idea that human beings have freedom of a personal will. This means that a person can produce a behavior by a conscious, intentional thought, through the action of some internal agent, even without control or influence by any condition of the environment. To be sure, personal freedom to choose behaviors is a necessary assumption of religion.

As the above descriptions indicate, only the Humanistic view of psychology is fully compatible with a religious orientation. That is not greatly surprising because the psychological theories were crafted to deal with the psychological, rather than the religious aspects of human beings. Indeed, the best that we can expect of a psychological theory is that it be compatible with religion. So, to produce a complete comprehensive view of the whole person, we must add appropriate religious concepts to a compatible psychological theory.

Humanistic psychology also emphasizes certain so-called human characteristics of persons. For example, it exalts the wholeness and uniqueness of human beings. It says that the whole person is healthy, productive and successful. Humanism also emphasizes that psychological events are often important only in terms of what they mean to, or have an impact on, the individual. And, finally, the responsibility for behavior can be personal rather than environmental, such that behavior is intentional and purposeful, instead of simply a mindless mechanical reaction to environmental cues. All these decidedly human characteristics help to make the Humanistic theory easily compatible with our religious beliefs.

Thus, the psychological theory of Humanism celebrates some particular human qualities of people, especially the possession of freedom of will. Nevertheless, it also deplores some of the human failings of people, those that prevent a person from becoming the best person that he or she might become. These presumptions about human beings are entirely consistent with a Christian model of people.

This book proposes therefore that we supplement our psychological theory of Humanism with religious concepts that will produce a more complete conception of human beings. The more complete conception of people allows us a fuller array of devices, remedies and therapies to enrich human life. The ultimate goal for the Christian is atonement with God. There can be no better condition for mental health.

Psychological Remedies and Therapies

The advocacy of Christian living suggests the ultimate in good psychotherapy, because the personal qualities that make for a good psychotherapist are the very characteristics of a good Christian. Indeed, the psychological evidence indicates clearly that the personal characteristics of the therapist are actually much more important to the success of a therapy than are the particular theories or methods that are adopted by that therapist. Moreover, in the context of certain kinds of psychotherapy, the expectations for the person in therapy are similar to those for the Christian who is striving for perfection in Christian living.

There are several kinds of psychological interventions, each based on certain assumptions about the nature of human beings and the nature of the underlying causation of the presenting problem. The psychological intervention is often identified as therapy, although the meaning of that term has been the subject of considerable debate. For example, the term can imply a curative or healing process as a remedy for a sickness. Psychologists do not like that connotation of the word. To be sure, we conventionally use the term "mental health," but we do not mean to imply that the lack of it is a sickness in the medical sense. To psychologists, mental health refers generally to a feeling of happiness and satisfaction in life, and confidence in a personal ability to cope with ordinary problems.

There are two basic approaches to restoring mental health of a person. One approach rests on the assumption that a person has some freedom to choose his or her behaviors, and the other does not. To avoid confusion, I will use the word "remedies" to refer to the processes of changing only behaviors and cognitions, and the term "insight therapies" to refer to the processes of helping people to change something about themselves personally, in a more fundamental way. It should be noted, however, that paradoxically the approaches that deny freedom of will often require the client to agree voluntarily to accept the help that is offered, in whatever form.[8]

Remedies

The technique of behavior modification is a remedy based solely on principles of learning. Therefore, it does not require the cooperation of the client, or any change of beliefs or attitudes. Because it merely involves evoked changes in overt behaviors, it is not very important here, except insofar as the selection of the target behaviors—by the therapist or mentor—is based on Christian goals.

Similarly, so-called behavior therapy is partly based on principles of learning, but it also incorporates target changes in beliefs and attitudes. So it is a hybrid therapy. Therefore, it is not truly a therapy according to the definition that I have given above because the clinician is not interested in changing the person, but in altering certain habits of behavior and thinking of that person. Nevertheless, the client must agree to accept the help.

Again, only the nature of the goals of treatment is particularly important with this method. A successful treatment removes an undesired behavior.

Insight Therapies

In the case of so-called insight therapies, the therapist attempts to foster some significant change in the stable personality characteristics of the person, not just in more or less superficial habits of thought and overt behaviors. There are three major categories of such insight therapies: Psychoanalysis, Cognitive Therapy and Humanistic Therapy. The first two are not directly relevant here because they both deny the existence of a human will which has a measure of freedom. But, ironically, with these views, as also true with behavior therapy, the client must make a voluntary choice just to submit to the therapeutic process.

The technique of psychoanalysis seeks to de-sensitize the client to certain personal pleasure-seeking impulses (i.e., "sex") that he or she had previously found threatening to his or her peace of mind, and thus caused personal anxiety. The resulting change in attitude in the client is produced by the therapeutic situation itself, and not by some conscious intention by the client.

The processes of cognitive therapy seek to change the beliefs and attitudes of the client by pointing out how his or her patterns of thinking are producing behaviors that are maladaptive. Again, the thought processes are changed by learning and cognitive mechanisms, without relying on the voluntary efforts of the client.

Humanistic therapy is an insight therapy based on the assumption of a conscious, voluntary effort of the client to achieve personal improvement. Thus, it is the only psychotherapy that is based on the theoretical assumption of a viable human will.

Actually, this approach to psychotherapy parallels, or mirrors, the practice of Christian religion. For example, the Humanistic therapy proposed by Rogers is based on three premises that closely approximate major tenets of Christianity: Genuineness, Empathy, and Unconditional Positive Regard for Others.[9]

To be genuine is to be exactly as you hold yourself out to be. You do not lie, misrepresent or dissemble. In particular, you do not fake positive attitudes or feelings for others because, for you, the feelings are real.

Empathy is to identify emotionally with another person. To be empathic is to feel the suffering and joy of another as if it were your own. Therefore, it goes beyond mere sympathy.

Unconditional positive regard means to accept, without reservation, another person as he or she is. It means to have good positive feelings for a person, regardless of how you feel about the attitudes and behaviors of that person. It is an approximation of the Christian concept of unearned love, or agape'.

Just as a religious counselor or pastor cannot give a person Christianity, a psychotherapist cannot give a person mental health. The therapist, like the pastor, is merely an advocate and an enabler, someone who helps the client in his or her quest. The therapist realizes—even asserts—that the improvement must come through the dedicated efforts of the client. With the grace of God, the client and the Christian deserve a significant portion of personal credit for his or her achievement of mental health.

Humanistic therapy is very much like the attempt of the Christian to achieve spiritual health. Basically, the same techniques of striving for peace of soul work for achieving peace of mind. In fact, I have gone so far as to assert that an essential part of psychotherapy is virtually identical to the establishment of a positive connection between a Christian and his or her friend or mentor.[10] Moreover, I submit that the Christian cannot achieve good mental health without also achieving spiritual health.

Convictions

I accept the traditional belief that each person's convictions about nature are primarily empirical, which means that they are produced in part by information about the physical world that is experienced in our minds through the use of our physical senses. This is in fact the conventional view that is held by psychologists, as well as the belief of the general public.

But, in addition, I believe also in an unorthodox view. I believe that our convictions are also molded by another kind of information about all things that is experienced in our minds by way of a direct process. This second process, initiated by God, does not require the eyes and ears, or indeed any other sensory system. It is surely first-person data.

This intuitive process is, to be sure, less well understood than the processing of empirical information. Indeed many psychologists—probably most of them—doubt that such a process even exists. Nevertheless, as a Christian and as a psychologist, I make three assertions in this respect: (1) both avenues for understanding the nature of the universe exist; (2) both avenues have been made available to us by God to help us understand Him and the universe that He has constructed; and (3) no one can disprove the first two assertions.

Our convictions about the world are therefore the result of a combination of the information that we have gained through both domains for gathering information—i.e., the sensory (empirical) and the non-sensory (intuitive or inspirational). Because both domains are equally valid, each of us must sift and process the information of both kinds, reaching some compatible convictions that are personally comfortable and workable. Because our information is necessarily incomplete, or is not fully understood, at some point the two domains of information may seem to conflict, and difficult decisions must be made concerning what to believe.

Sometimes, we must simply postpone judgment until, hopefully, we finally understand the available information. Often, we cannot do that. Then, we must adopt the conclusion that seems best. In this connection, I have proposed what I call the Principle of Ultimate Practicality, as follows: "In the absence of clear empirical or logical proof to the contrary, each individual person may conditionally believe whatever seems to work most harmoniously and effectively to achieve personal goals and to promote personal growth."[11] This psychological principle is a practical rule for the guidance of individual behavior. It means that logically every person is free to believe anything that is not contradicted by convincing proof, empirical or logical, if that belief truly works to make him or her effective and happy in daily living—i.e., promotes mental health. I believe that Christian truths belong in this category.

Thus, we surely accept as true the psychological principles in the Bible that science has convincingly verified. But, this generalization says that we can also believe principles that work—make sense—for us even though they have not been proved by science. This principle removes the burden to prove each of our convictions scientifically.

I emphatically do *not* believe that any principles in the Bible have ever been *disproved* by science. Apparent disproof appears only because of literal misinterpretations of the true literary and poetic language that is characteristic of the Bible.

The Principle of Ultimate Practicality also means that a person is *not* free to disbelieve that which *has* been proved by science. For example, a conviction that the law of gravity is false will not work for the benefit of anyone. To step off a high roof into open space will undeniably produce adverse consequences.

It would be equally foolish to reject a proven medical treatment on the grounds that such treatment was not of God. Such an idea is preposterous and actually blasphemous. Although, admittedly, a specific treatment may not be mentioned in the Bible, the Bible does assure us, as we have said, that everything that was made was created by the hand of God. To be sure, we can encounter an ethical decision about whether or not a given treatment represents the loving response in a particular situation, but that is an entirely different matter. Just as the writing of the Bible was divinely inspired, the discovery of scientific laws was divinely inspired. Therefore, the Christian is not forced to make a choice between them.

One caveat is important: we must understand that any scientific law entails a small seed for doubt. Statements of laws are crafted as an act of human wisdom. Therefore, logically we must admit that new evidence could require that we modify a previously accepted physical law.

So, we must live with some doubts about the lesser details of life on this earth. But, for health and happiness, we must hold to some convictions about the realities of life, which then control our behaviors.

While we must understand the limitations of scientific inquiry, and the multifarious problems of interpreting scientific data, we must not discount scientific facts. Unfortunately, some religionists attempt to do just that. For example, an ordained minister once said in my hearing, "There are no facts, only perceptions." His assertion proves that different people can read the same Bible, but do not necessarily agree on what it is saying. When God made this world, He also made truth, and thus facts. Ironically, the cleric was misled probably by some casual contact with the modernity view of science, which emphasizes an element of intrinsic subjectivity in science. To be sure, such subjectivity must be considered. But, the modernity view does not deny the existence of stubborn facts, which are objective facts, ones that hold up despite the wishes and views of the different observers of those facts.

A wise God would not establish a chaotic world in which the only truth was the immediate subjective experience of the individual observer. The implications of such a world are indeed frightening. For example, there could be no justice, because only the perception of the powerful would matter. There could be no comfort from awareness of the consistency produced by knowledge of an orderly world. We could not function if one person's fact were likely to be another person's fiction.

To be sure, the existence of truth provides an intersection or overlapping of science and religion. Truth is the primary goal of science. It is second only to love as a goal of the Christian religion. When the welfare of a person is involved, truth is an essential consequence of love. It is not possible to love someone, and deliberately fabricate, accept or ignore a falsehood to them or about them.

No one can remember exactly in all cases just where his or her personal convictions originated. We have had the benefits of the knowledge and thoughts of many teachers and preachers, families and friends, who helped to shape our views. Nevertheless, each of us, ourselves, must take responsibility for the beliefs that we have ultimately accepted, and for the actions that stem from them.

Value of Convictions

I pray that the observations and conclusions in this book will be useful to empower the readers in the further development of their own beliefs and their abilities to serve. Thus, I hope to increase their power to live by the faith that they have adopted and developed by their personal efforts. The development of this individual faith is the beginning of a happier life. It marks the acceptance of Jesus Christ as our bridge to God, and thus to enjoy the fruits of His love.

As the keynote messages tell us, improvement in personal welfare comes from committing one's life to something truly important, rather than to selfish needs. Therefore, wisdom is revealed in its very uses. As James said, true wisdom of the mind is revealed by the performance of good deeds:

> Who is wise and understanding among you? Let him show it by his good life, by deeds done in the humility that comes from wisdom. But if you harbor bitter envy and selfish ambition in your hearts, do not boast about it or deny the truth. Such "wisdom" does not come down from heaven but is earthly, unspiritual, of the devil. For where you have envy and selfish ambition, there you find disorder and every evil practice.
>
> But the wisdom that comes from heaven is first of all pure; then peace-loving, considerate, submissive, full of mercy, and good fruit, impartial and sincere. Peacemakers who sow in peace raise a harvest of righteousness.[12]

Such is the power that can be unleashed by understanding the Holy Bible. You can use your own mind and spirit to incorporate that power in your life.

Others may help, but in the end only you can release this power for yourself.

This book maintains that the practice of religion is the ultimate method of psychotherapy, both for yourself and for others about you. While endorsing the appropriate and sensible uses of the technologies that have been developed by psychological science, the book strongly asserts that, particularly for the health of society, these technologies must be used with a psychotherapeutic frame of mind and with the right spirit of selfless service. Without the Holy Spirit, the bare technologies will not save our society.

Virtue vs. Conformity

A person has virtue to the extent that he or she is committed to acting on the basis of Christian convictions. This basis of behavior stands in sharp contradiction to merely moral behavior in which a person simply conforms to the rules or standards of behavior for a given group of people.

Norms are the usual behaviors of the group. They are discovered by simple observations, whether those observations are made by behavioral scientists, or by individual persons for themselves. Norms can become the basis of rules of behavior, which, if followed, can be used to justify the individual. The idea of justifying oneself by following rules is called legalism, a term which is abhorred by Christians. For Christians, always the spirit counts more than the rules.

Norms of group behavior are not necessarily based on Christian principles. Because the possession of virtue is the key to the door of a happy life, conformity to the normal behaviors of a group does not guarantee happiness. A person cannot wrap himself or herself in a cloak of virtue in order to achieve happiness. Therefore, a person should not try to be virtuous because that stance in this world is practical. God's laws do not work in such a mechanical, superficial way. Nothing works without the initial acceptance of God and a commitment to Him. Without such commitment, the person is merely trying to conform to the observed behaviors of the people called Christians. That is moral, but it is not virtuous. For example, the physical act of joining a church or other religious group is moral behavior, but it is not necessarily virtuous.

It is the deeds of virtuous living that are the ones of practical value in building a better life for the individual, and a more peaceful world. In fact, I have asserted previously that such spiritual thinking is essential to the very survival of our human society on this planet.[13] The same conclusion has been reached by many other psychologists and social observers. Science can stop short of God, but scientists must not.

Notes

1. John B. Watson, Psychology as the Behaviorist views it. *Psychological Review,* 20, (1913), 158-177.
2. Sigmund Freud. *An Outline of Psychoanalysis*, trans. J. Strachey (New York: Norton, 1949).
3. Carl R. Rogers, A theory of therapy, personality, and interpersonal relationships, as developed in the client-centered framework. In *Psychology: A Study of a Science,* Vol. 3, ed. Sigmund Koch (New York: McGraw-Hill, 1954), 184-256.
4. Watson, Psychology as the Behaviorist views it.
5. Donald O. Hebb, *The Organization of Behavior* (New York: Wiley, 1949).
6. Watson, Psychology as the Behaviorist views it, Burrhus F. Skinner, *Science and Human Behavior* (New York: McMillan, 1953).
7. Hebb, *The Organization of Behavior;* Jean Piaget, *The Child's Conception of the World* (New York: Harcourt, Brace, 1929). Freud, *An Outline of Psychoanalysis*; Rogers, A theory of therapy; Abraham H. Maslow, Humanistic science and transcendental experiences, *Journal of Humanistic Psychology,* 5, (1965), 219-227.
8. E. Rae Harcum, Barry N. Burijon and Neill Watson, Client responsibility in the practitioner's operational definition of behavior therapy. *Journal of Human Behavior and Learning,* 5, (1988), 12-16.
9. Rogers, A theory of therapy.
10. E. Rae Harcum, *The Incidental Psychotherapy in Christian Connection.* (unpublished manuscript).
11. E. Rae Harcum, *A Psychology of Freedom and Dignity* (Westport, CT: Praeger, 1994), 38.
12. Holy Bible, New International Version (Grand Rapids, MI: Zondervan Publishing House, 1973), James 3: 13-18.
13. Harcum, *A Psychology of Freedom and Dignity.*

PART II. GOD'S LOVE

Chapter 3

The Call

We surely pay a heavy price when we disobey God's laws, and fail to behave responsibly and to love. The proof is around us. Consider the sorry state of our society, which we have helped to create. Anyone who is inclined to doubt this sad assertion is referred to the daily newspaper, the newscasts or to the talk shows on television. The stresses and dangers of modern life reach into every home and community, such that no one is unaffected. Therefore, no one can be truly peaceful and happy until everyone can share in a better society, despite grand individual plans for personal well-being. Religion is the pathway to this better society. Our sick society desperately needs a revival of Christian thinking and action for the benefit of all people.

Desperate calls for remedial social action, coming from many varied sources, have been undeniably clear. For example, in a speech commemorating the 300th anniversary of the Sir Christopher Wren Building at The College of William and Mary, the president of the university, Timothy J. Sullivan, starkly described the problems facing our world, as follows:

> We have spawned a popular culture that should shame a civilized people. Its avidity for violence, its exaltation of vulgarity and selfishness, reflect a sickness of spirit which we must quickly cure or face the fatal consequences.
>
> Our public discourse has likewise been coarsened and corrupted. Political debate—debate is too kind a word—is dominated by noisy, self-certain partisans at either end of the philosophical spectrum. The sensible center has fallen largely silent while the true believers of the right and of the left conduct a rhetorical war that consists largely of exchanging angry shouts. Backing up both sides are masters of the blackest political arts—skilled manipulators whose most distinctive quality is their cynicism and whose greatest talent is for clever character assassination.[1]

Surely, no thinking citizen would dispute Sullivan's crisp conclusion about the pervasiveness of our social problems. And surely no one would doubt the need for an early solution to those problems. This truly is our mission as Christians.

Pathway to a Solution

Social observers of the problems have suggested solutions, many grounded on virtuous thinking. For example, Sullivan himself suggested old-fashioned virtues as a general path toward the solution of our social ills:

> May I suggest that the answer lies not in an effusion of new prescriptions from crackpot ideologies safely cocooned in their Washington think tanks? More helpful by far would be the fresh recollection of old virtues which were so clearly controlling in the lives of those who built the College and watched this building rise brick by brick.[2]

Sullivan listed some of those redeeming virtues for the citizens in a healthy society: selflessness, honor, faith, decency and a commitment to constructive collaborative work for the good of all. Social improvement naturally follows such improvements in personal outlooks and lifestyles.

Such desired virtues are indeed part of a Christian life. A key ingredient is a love and caring for the welfare of others. For example, Jesus was asked which of the commandments is the most important:

> 'The most important one,' answered Jesus, 'is this: Hear, O Israel, the Lord our God, the Lord is one. Love the Lord your God with all your heart and with all your soul and with all your mind and with all your strength. The second is this: Love your neighbor as yourself. There is no commandment greater than these.'[3]

Jesus' answer was at once a call for us to solve the problems of society, and a blueprint for the solution. We must increase our commitment to love. The closest psychological term for this solution is "Unconditional Positive Regard," a major component in Humanistic psychotherapy.[4]

A similar call has come from psychiatry. For example, the psychiatric approach of Reality Therapy, developed by William Glasser, argues that psychiatry must deal with two basic human needs: *"the need to love and be loved and the need to feel that we are worthwhile to ourselves and to others."*[5] Glasser argues that some people can fill these needs without religion, while others cannot feel worthwhile unless religion is an integral part of their lives. The individual person must decide which path is best for him or for her.

Irresponsible people do not behave in ways that satisfy these personal needs. The function of a Reality Therapist is to teach responsible methods to people in order to satisfy their needs. As Glasser said, "Our job is not to lessen the pain of irresponsible actions, but to increase the patient's strength so that he can bear the necessary pain of a full life as well as enjoy the rewards of a deeply responsible existence."[6] To be sure, triumphant living does not imply a complete absence of pain, but a series of victories over temptations. Glasser emphasized that his therapy entailed a central role for the teaching of ethical values as a part of responsible behavior.

Modern religious writers concur. For example, Clark Morphew, an ordained clergyman and religious columnist, cited a study by the Heritage Foundation of Washington, D.C., which concluded that there are numerous positive personal and social benefits from a regular practice of religion. Morphew concluded:

> All you have to do is get into the habit of regular religious practice. And if we all did that, this country would be so much better we would think we were living in the vestibule of heaven.
> I believe illegal drug use would go down along with crimes of all kinds. Families would stay intact and children would grow up with a stronger moral foundation. Eventually gangs would disappear and we could walk without fear.[7]

A similar view was stated by William Raspberry, columnist for the *Washington Post*.[8] Raspberry quoted Robert Woodson, the founder and President of the National Center for Neighborhood Enterprise in Washington, D.C., as saying that the successful programs for social welfare in the inner cities almost always include a "spiritual element." Although spiritual does not necessarily mean religious, it does include the basic virtues in religion: a commitment to other people and an unconditional caring for them. These virtues give meaning to the life of the youth in the inner city.

These social programs work because, as Raspberry concluded, the fundamental problem causing bad behavior is the woeful lack of training in the social virtues of our young people. He said:

> It is simply another manifestation of a problem I have described as the "consciencelessness" of a small but significant element among us: children who have reached adolescence and beyond without having internalized any important sense of right and wrong, who have no internal brakes on their behavior, who can maim, destroy and kill without remorse.[9]

Raspberry proposes a solution, as follows: "And we can do what is necessary to reduce at the source the supply of conscienceless youngsters—*by enlisting church and community in a crusade, for their academic, economic and spiritual redemption*" (emphasis added).[10] Therefore, the message is again the familiar one: the church and religious leaders must help to supply the spiritual element in any rehabilitation program for the members of society.

This long-range view is further supported by Joan Beck, also a columnist and social observer, who asserts: "And we must try to strengthen and expand the positive influences in our society, *particularly the churches*, whose moral values are the necessary foundation of our society, whether or not they are so acknowledged" (emphasis added).[11] In my view, we are too often distracted from these obviously beneficial ethical influences by focusing on the secondary issues of abortion and homosexuality.

Finally, Tony Snow, a syndicated columnist with the *Detroit News*, commenting on the assertion of Gov. Jesse Ventura of Minnesota that religion is a crutch for weak minds, said, "Of course religion is a crutch. Without it, civilization collapses—but so do the common-sense virtues Ventura espoused on the campaign trail."[12] Snow argued that some things are absolutely right or absolutely wrong, regardless of who is in power. Martyrs who are strong-minded enough to die for their beliefs protect the rights of us all, and thus preserve the society. He concluded, "If you dispense with religion, you abandon the central tenet of our democracy—that all people possess inalienable rights. Justice becomes a matter for leaders to decide. Dignity becomes a luxury; not a birthright."[13]

So, the right message is indeed out there: The deeds of virtuous people are needed. We Christians must join in supplying the vital spiritual element that is required for successful social programs. Christians—notably within the churches—must accept and assume their central role of leadership in turning our youth back to basic Judeo-Christian virtues.

Many times Jesus commanded that we take His spirit of love into the world. His language cannot be misunderstood. But, sadly, the sordid madness that has taken over so much of our society today provides compelling evidence that too few church members have faithfully followed His bidding. In an earlier draft of this book, I used the term "professed Christians" to identify lukewarm members of the church. I stopped using the term because it is either a redundancy or an oxymoron. It is a redundancy because a Christian is naturally called upon to witness, to profess Christianity. The term is an oxymoron if the person verbally professes Christ, but does not follow His commandments.

Admittedly, I do not have a totally satisfactory term. The term "hypocrite" does not capture the full flavor of what I have in mind. Therefore, for convenience, I have now settled on the term "tinsel lover." The term was suggested to me by a humorous line attributed to the late Oscar Levant, a film star and humorist. In describing Hollywood, Levant said that under all of the tinsel and glitter, there was pure tinsel and glitter. So it is with the tinsel lover in the church: under all of the form of a religion, there is pure pomp and circumstance. Thus, the so-called "tinsel lover" in the church manifests some of the outward behaviors of a Christian, specifically the overt profession of faith. Such behaviors dress up the person like tinsel decorates a Christmas tree. But, the value goes no deeper.

We are familiar with instances of convicted felons professing to be born-again Christians in the hope of receiving lighter sentences for their crimes. Judge Russell Carneal cited the case of a defendant who threw his allegedly cherished Bible against a courtroom wall after he received a maximum sentence.[14]

The tinsel description refers specifically to those who profess Christ, but largely ignore particularly the second half of His Great Commandment. God's plan includes a place for us to assist in the building of His kingdom. Peter used the image of living stones to convey this message:

> As you come to him, the living Stone—rejected by men but chosen by God by God and precious to him—you also, like living stones, are being built into a spiritual house to be a holy priesthood, offering spiritual sacrifices acceptable to God through Jesus Christ.[15]

But we have not acted like living stones for the construction of a spiritual house. Morphew blames primarily the church leaders for failing to mount an effective defense, or counterattack, against the forces in our society that attack religion and glorify ungodly activities. He calls such activities as sex and violence in the movies and television "the trashing of moral values in this country."[16] These same media, commissioned to dispense information and entertainment for the public good, seldom present a positive view of religious faith. That destructive tendency should be attacked with our utmost efforts.

Morphew answered the question of how we restore the influence of religion in our daily lives:

> That's easy. We do religion. We participate in worship. We stop carping about our leader's wrinkled suit and we get behind a national effort to rebuild a spiritual presence in our neighborhoods.
> And we hit the streets with the religious message of our choice. Take your faith to the people. I believe we will feel better, and so will the nation.[17]

Indeed, God's charge to us is for spiritual revival. But, some modern churches do not even like to talk about revival. Nevertheless, Jesus made the charge to revival totally clear in the church in Matthew:

> You are the salt of the earth. But if the salt loses its saltiness, how can it be made salty again? It is no longer good for anything, except to be thrown out and trampled by men.
> You are the light of the world. A city on a hill cannot be hidden. Neither do people light a lamp and put it under a bowl. Instead they put it on its stand, and it gives light to everyone in the house. In the same way, let your light shine before men, that they may see your good deeds and praise your Father in heaven.[18]

I have also used the term, Churchian, to refer to persons in the church with tinsel-loving characteristics.[19] A Churchian is a member of a church who professes Christ but loves the church building and organization more than he or she loves Christ. The point here is that the purported Christian's words of devotion are hollow and meaningless unless they are validated by acts of love and service to others.

This book encourages committed Christians to increase their participation and service in the daily functioning of the world, and to do it in a way that glorifies their faith. To aid in this vital Christian responsibility, the book offers spiritual enrichment from the Bible, supplemented by psychological tools. The mental health of everyone will be improved as the world becomes a place of love, truth, trust and peace.

The Psychological Tools

As I have discussed elsewhere, a psychological plan for the survival of our society must be based on psychotherapeutic principles, rather than on impersonal technological advances in behavioral science.[20] Indeed, the problems of society are caused by flaws in personalities. As Sullivan was quoted above, the antisocial behaviors are but symptoms of disordered personalities.[21] The bare technologies focus on changing the behaviors, but deliberately ignore the need to change the people. Such an approach violates the first psychological principle of good problem solving: Identify the actual factor or factors that are blocking the attainment of the goal. If the true problem is not identified, it cannot be solved, despite a flurry of dedicated activity and promises of good intentions.

In sum, the important problems in our society are the antisocial attitudes and beliefs that form the core personalities of the people. Persons who devote their lives to achieving personal satisfactions and happiness can never be fundamentally satisfied and happy. We must change the people.

At this point, I emphasize that the blending of spiritual and psychological tools for self-improvement will work not only to bring psychological peace directly to the individuals in society, but also indirectly to the society as a whole. As John Donne wrote in his classic poem, no man is an island. Therefore, whenever we make life better for someone else, we thereby improve the psychological climate for our own lives. Not only do we ourselves grow spiritually and psychologically from helping others, we also benefit from their improved behaviors toward us.

Personal Commitments

There are two separate, but interrelated, faces of the Christian's total commitment. The Christian will recognize the two faces from the two parts of the Great Commandment given to us by Jesus: to love God; and to love our neighbors as ourselves. The first face is vital to the personal salvation of the individual Christian. The second face assumes that the second part of the commandment—to love one's neighbor—will follow as a natural consequence if the first is fully understood and faithfully obeyed. This social face is vital to the survival of the human society in which the Christian lives. I submit that a society without Christian practices will die. To be sure, these behaviors can be practiced by non-Christians, but they cannot be sustained and endure through inevitable trials, if they are not rooted in a belief in the one true God, as revealed in Jesus Christ.

An examination of the second face actually tells us whether or not we have understood and followed the first part of the Commandment. It tries to help us understand what specific behaviors in the second face indicate that we truly have been loving God with our whole hearts, minds and strengths. We need such guidance because our sheer desire to follow the Christian path does not ensure that we will actually make the right choices.[22] No one practices his or her Christianity in a world without people. We are constantly reminded in the Scriptures that the love of God necessarily requires care and concern for His people.

This necessity for the tangible manifestation of love is made clear at many points in the Bible. For example, James, brother of Jesus, writing to all Christians, said:

> What good is it, my brothers if a man claims to have faith but has no deeds? Can such faith save him? Suppose a brother or sister is without clothes and daily food. If one of you says to him, 'Go, I wish you well; keep warm and well fed,' but does nothing about his physical needs, what good is it? In the same way, faith by itself, if it is not accompanied by action, is dead.
> But someone will say, 'You have faith; I have deeds.'
> Show me your faith without deeds, and I will show you my faith by what I do. . . . As the body without the spirit is dead so faith without deeds is dead.[23]

Henderson and Casper would agree. Their book is a running dialogue between a pastor (Jim) and an atheist (Casper) as they visit various churches about the country. After Casper attended a church service in the home of a Christian friend, Jason, he remarked that he sincerely respected Jason and his friends, even though he did not share their beliefs. Jim asked how Casper differentiated between Christians that he respected and those that he did not respect. Casper responded:

> Jason doesn't have a big church or a million bucks or ten trips to Africa under his belt, but I see firsthand—almost every time we speak or get together—that he walks the walk.
> He helps African immigrants find their way around town. He and his wife teach English as a second language. He helps people build their homes (case in point: the kickboards in my house that I could in no way have installed without his help). He regularly opens his home to others. And he does it all because of his belief that Jesus is his Lord, and for him, this is what Jesus would have done.[24]

As the words of Casper imply, our good deeds reveal what is in our hearts. The faith of theology and the science of psychology entirely agree on this fundamental consistency between the basic personality characteristics of an individual and his or her overt behaviors. Sometimes, because of outside pressures there is a discrepancy between beliefs and actions, to be sure, but ordinarily they are consistent. An inconsistency makes the person feel uncomfortable, and therefore causes him or her to change either the actions or the beliefs to bring them into agreement.

The Personal Face

Psychological research shows that Christians who actually practice their religion will personally enjoy better mental health.[25] Therefore, making Christian choices involves a no-lose situation, personally as well as for the general society.

To be sure, all Christians have made the most important choice, perhaps many years before, in deciding to follow Jesus. But, we have been forced by circumstances every day since that original religious conversion to re-affirm that decision for Christ in our daily lives. Daily we must make choices toward Christian goals, or toward sinful paths. Too often, we do not have a conscious awareness of just what is at stake in that particular decision. We do not understand that an evil path that we have chosen actually amounts to a denial of Christ. Tragically, we assume that, because we were "saved" at some point in our lives, all of our decisions are naturally and necessarily Christian. This conclusion is a natural inference from the assertion of Blackaby and King that, because God works through Christians, their behaviors are His behaviors.[26] Although that may not be what these authors intend to say, this assertion implies that a human being could actually respond with perfection. I do not understand the Bible to be saying anything of the sort. We will be good *if* we choose atonement with God.

Sometimes, we even deliberately take the un-Christian path, even though we know that it is wrong. To do so is to take God's forgiveness for granted. I have serious doubt that God works by that plan, because He is a jealous God.

Because life situations usually differ, the task of the Christian is to know how to apply the truths of his or her religion to particular situations. Indeed, the principles for guidance cannot be foolproof prescriptions for ethical behaviors to be used blindly or indiscriminately whenever some ethical dilemma appears. As Marty warned:

> No one has the sole key to the ways that religion and the public should meet in a kinetic, pluralist society. The mix is too rich, the set of situations is too volatile, and the repository of plausible proposals from many sources is too well-stocked to permit anyone's sense of having arrived at full resolutions.[27]

Thus, the best way to prepare for Christian living is to develop a Christian outlook, to develop a Christian conscience by which many good behaviors can be generated and evaluated. The reader is urged to read this book reflectively, to look for messages and insights. This approach is better than seeking simple rules to follow that purportedly will ensure perfect responses under all conditions and in all situations.

The healthy conscience does not preclude the continuing need for evaluating our decisions. Just as there is the capacity for good in every sinner, there is the capacity to sin in every human being, including Christians. Remember that Jesus had high praise for the tax collector who acknowledged his sinfulness, and condemnation for the Pharisee who reveled in his own presumed righteousness. This book is not intended to make Christians feel proud of themselves. It is intended to make Christians feel good about their victories against temptations to sin.

This book may well not contain the answer to a specific problem for anyone. I hope that it can help some readers craft satisfactory Christian answers for themselves for the important occasions when they need good answers.

Help in making Christian decisions comes in two forms. The first is simply to boost the motivation to be Christ-like. The second is to improve the ability to distinguish Christian choices from unchristian ones. The Bible helps as the basic source of guidance. We believe in the inerrancy of the Bible, to be sure. We cannot be as sure of our ability to interpret the Bible accurately in order to guide our actions in the specific cases that confront us, as I have said before.[28] For example, the Bible literally tells us not to owe anything to any man. We can conclude therefore that it prohibits the purchase of anything on credit. Or, we can interpret the same passage as telling us to pay our bills on time. The latter interpretation seems more reasonable. I just cannot think that taking out a mortgage on a house is sinful. But, I can easily view the deliberate failure to make mortgage payments—or child-support payments, etc.—as patently sinful.

A specific pertinent example of possible misinterpretation of the Bible is the admonition to be calm. The Bible says to trust that God will take care of you. This could be taken as instructions simply to fold your arms and relax, waiting for God's blessings of peace to descend. But, I think that this interpretation is the exception to a more reasonable principle, indicated by other passages in the Bible. Often, the people of God are chided for inaction, for failure to use their talents. Jesus cursed the unproductive fig tree, clearly involving metaphor. This passage tells us that we too should be productive. So, God wants you to be sufficiently concerned in order to take positive action in the world. He promises us peace if we trust in Him as we work. His promise gives us courage and confidence to labor in His vineyards.

The reader must incorporate these ideas into his or her personal life, in order to be able to use them in extremely personal decisions. These decisions may be entirely private. At other times, they may also be displayed in relationships with others—in the home, in the church, in the workplace and at play. Thus , as Marty said, religion has, on the one hand, a private face that speaks to the inner needs of the people. He said: "Religion has to speak to them in the long night watches, in times of private terror and personal joy, or it will not speak to them at all."[29]

The Social Face

This same religion must also hold up in the crucible of public life. Therefore, Marty also said: "The test of faith is under the light of public interchange, and the achievement of religion must include a reasonably successful encounter in the marketplace, the forum of ideas, the arena where human suffering is most visible, where the demand for service is greatest."[30] Although a religion of love can comfort the personal soul, it will permit no rest in the face of suffering by neighbors.

Making Christian decisions requires personal power, both spiritual and psychological, which cannot be found in mere lists of rules to follow. Jesus made this point clear in the familiar story of the rich young ruler:

> A certain ruler asked him, 'Good teacher, what must I do to inherit eternal life?'
> 'Why do you call me good?' Jesus answered. 'No one is good—except God alone. You know the commandments: 'Do not commit adultery, do not murder, do not steal, do not give false testimony, honor your father and mother.'
> 'All these I have kept since I was a boy,' he said.
> When Jesus heard this, he said to him, 'You still lack one thing. Sell everything you have and give to the poor, and you will have treasure in heaven. Then come, follow me.'
> When he heard this, he became very sad, because he was a man of great wealth. Jesus looked at him and said, 'How hard it is for the rich to enter the kingdom of God! Indeed, it is easier for a camel to go through the eye of a needle than for a rich man to enter the kingdom of God.'[31]

Thus, the power to be good is not the power to adhere to rules. For example, the effectiveness of a psychotherapist is related more to the good personal characteristics and style of the therapist than to the particular theory and nominal therapeutic techniques that the therapist adopts. Similarly, the style of leadership employed by the supervisor—e.g., authoritarian vs. egalitarian— is less important than whether the supervisor communicates to his or her workers an attitude of caring for their welfare.

Indeed, the power for positive change must come from the inner resources of the virtuous person. These inner resources include strong Christian beliefs, the commitment to act on those beliefs and the knowledge and skills to translate those Christian characteristics into successful service and witness to our neighbors. The Scriptures thus indicate that the rich young ruler was really not a virtuous person. We know this because he went away sorrowing at the news that simple adherence to established church rules was not sufficient for a Christian, and consequently not sufficient to inherit eternal life.

Discussion

The present book is intended to empower the reader to make the Christian selection when he or she is confronted with the complex and confusing decisions of living in the modern world. But, the author does not—and indeed cannot —

guarantee success. Triumphant living ultimately depends upon the empowered decisions by the individual Christian.

I have always been intrigued by some people who profess to know what is the proper Christian response in every situation that poses a problem to Christian living. To me, life has always seemed far too complicated to permit pre-packaged answers to its serious problems. My years of psychological training and experience support this important fundamental truth.

To be sure, my commitment to love other people does not always lead me to know exactly what is the most ethical, the most loving, the psychologically most appropriate, response for me to make at a given time in a particular situation. This book assumes that many other Christians also have the same kinds of problems, despite their desires to be good Christians. They have trouble in deciding exactly what *is* the Christian response in particular situations that may require them to make ethical decisions.[32]

Jesus Himself avoided giving specific answers. Like any good teacher, He would not be trapped into giving precise rules. He answered direct questions with parables, or even with other pointed questions. He wanted to force the questioner to develop his or her own answers. For example, in Luke 10:23, Jesus answered the lawyer's question concerning the definition of a neighbor with the parable of the good Samaritan.[33] Then, He followed with the question about which of the three fellow travelers was neighbor to him who fell among the thieves. The correct answer was obvious from the basic meaning of the story. Therefore, Jesus wants us to have full spiritual and psychological understanding in order to enable us to find the correct answers for ourselves. Such is the technique of a master teacher.

The fullness of the discovered understanding means that the true message then becomes part of our personal belief systems, and thus we become virtuous persons. When these personal beliefs about life become incorporated into our daily behaviors, we have answered God's call.

Notes

1. Timothy J. Sullivan, Wren building stands as a symbol of college's vitality. *William and Mary News,* 25 (2), September 1, 1995, 5.
2. *ibid.*
3. Holy Bible, New International Version (Grand Rapids, MI: Zondervan Publishing House, 1973), Mark 12:29-31.
4. Carl R. Rogers, A theory of therapy, personality, and interpersonal relationships, as developed in the client-centered framework. In *Psychology: A Study of a Science,* Vol. 3, ed. Sigmund Koch (New York: McGraw-Hill, 1959), 184-256.
5. William Glasser, *Reality Therapy* (New York: Harper & Row, 1965), 10.
6. *ibid*, 72
7. Clark Morphew, Religion must hit the streets to change U. S. attitudes. *Daily Press*, Newport News, VA, February 23, 1996, D3.
8. William Raspberry, Make communities safe from and for children. *Daily Press*, Newport News, VA, August 19, 1994.
9. Raspberry, Make communities safe, A12.
10. *ibid.*
11. Joan Beck, The frustrating job of ending a culture of violence. *Daily Press*, Newport News, VA, September 10, 1994, A8.
12. Tony Snow, Ventura lost out with God. *Daily Press*, Newport News, VA, October 11, 1999, A15.
13. *ibid.*
14. Russel M. Carneal, Ethics of a jurist. In *Biblical Guidance and Human Choices*, ed. E. Rae Harcum (Williamsburg, VA: Cape Books, 1999), 222-239.
15. Holy Bible, 1 Peter 2: 4-5.
16. Morphew, Religion must hit the streets: D3.
17. *ibid.*
18. Holy Bible, Matthew 5: 13-16.
19. E. Rae Harcum, *Saving Our Church: Five Systemic Diseases Pose a Vital Mission for the Organized Church* (Lanham, MD: Hamilton Books, 2009).
20. E. Rae Harcum, *A Psychology of Freedom and Dignity*, (Westport, CT: Praeger, 1994). E. Rae Harcum, Implications of the Contradictions in Behaviorism for a Scientifically-Based Public Policy. In *The Integration of Psychological Principles in Policy Development*, ed. Chris E. Stout (Westport, CT: Praeger, 1995), 173-183.
21. Sullivan, Wren building stands as symbol.
22. E. Rae Harcum, ed. *Biblical Guidance and Human Choices*. (Williamsburg, VA: Cape Books. 1999).
23. Holy Bible, James 2:14-17.

24. Jim Henderson and Matt Casper, *Jim and Casper go to Church: Frank Conversations about Faith, Churches, and Well-meaning Christians* (Carol Stream, IL: Barna Books, 2007), 76.
25. J. F. Schumaker , ed., *Religion and Mental Health* (New York: Oxford University Press, 1992); W. Laurance Ventis, The relationships between religion and mental health. *Journal of Social Issues,* 5 (2), (1992), 33-48.
26. Henry T. Blackaby and C. V. King, *Experiencing God* (Nashville, TN: Broadman & Holman Publishers, 1994).
27. M. E. Marty, Foreword. In *Religion and American Public Life*, ed. R. W. Lovin. (New York: Paulist Press, 1986), 4.
28. Harcum, *Biblical Guidance.*
29. Marty, foreword: 1.
30. *ibid.*
31. Holy Bible, Luke 18: 18-25.
32. Harcum, *Biblical Guidance.*
33. Holy Bible, Luke 10: 23-37.

Chapter 4

Hearing The Message

The best advice for a Christian who would help a friend to achieve mental health would be, first, to become the best Christian that he or she could be. This chapter suggests ways for the Christian to become a better Christian.

The principles of psychology help us to focus and to organize our efforts toward achieving our Christian goals. Psychology advocates a system of orderly steps or stages in problem solving, as follows: (1) Establish a clear understanding of what is desired; (2) Craft and evaluate possible solutions; and (3) Try the different solutions in a reasonable order until you find one that satisfies the goal. The general process is much like constructing a map to reach an identified destination, with indicated landmarks along the way to help the traveler decide whether or not he or she is on the right track.

The desired goals of the Christian are explicitly stated by Paul in I Corinthians 13:13: "And now these three remain: faith, hope and love. But the greatest of these is love."[1] So, again, our first goal must be to love. Our problem as Christians—and as lay psychologists—is in finding and choosing the correct path to the sub-goal of overt manifestations of our love. In the confusing world around us, we cannot always tell which is the actual specific behavior that is most reflective of our inner love, and benefits the recipient the most. As is well known, good intentions do not guarantee a good result. Perseverance is not wonderful if the behavior itself is not loving.

The rest of this chapter, as well as essentially the remainder of this book, discusses possible solutions to finding the necessary pathway, or specific behaviors, to the expression of Christian love to those in our world about us. Thus, our task, as committed Christians, is to discover just how God's communications to us can be translated into specific actions in today's world. As I have discussed previously, the Bible is our guide, but it still does not obviate our need to make good decisions.[2]

Sometimes the translation of love into behaviors is easy. In such cases, we may need only the courage and good sense to do what we know that we should do. But, sometimes the selection of the Christian response is extremely difficult. In fact, Christians do not always agree on which behavior is best in a given situation. Therefore, each person must do his or her best to find behaviors that work. If an attempted solution does not work, we try others until we find one that does satisfy.

Forms of the Map

God guides us to our destination using combinations of five different methods, as follows: (1) The Bible; (2) Human witnesses; (3) Practical feedback; (4) Prayer/inspiration; and (5) Reasoning. If we do not fully understand His message in one form of instruction, we may respond better to an alternate form. These avenues to understanding are, of course, not mutually exclusive, but supportive of one another.

The Bible

The Bible provides us with God's instructions, and an earthly model of them in action in the expressed character and reported behaviors of Jesus. But, to be sure, there had to be a translation from the original foreign language. Recently, there have been newer translations into more modern forms. Therefore, the experts obviously concluded that the earlier language could be made clearer to us in terms of our particular experience.

Thus, the Bible presents God's message physically in words. We are verbal creatures and we tend to think in words. Nevertheless, frequently there are semantic problems in verbal communication. For example, the same words do not always mean exactly the same thing to different people, particularly if the different people have been brought up in different cultures, in different times and otherwise have had different experiences in life. For example, the English word "gay" has a vastly different connotation today than when I was a young man.

We may argue about whether a particular personal style is "assertive" or "pushy." The connotation of the first word in our society· is likely to be praiseworthy, while the other is not. In terms of the behavior, a normal degree of assertiveness in one social group may be considered too aggressive by another group.

Then, too, we may understand different meanings of words depending upon our particular perspective at the time. Therefore, we argue about the specific meanings of such terms as "flexible" and "capricious," as represented by a given behavior. Often, as we say, the meaning "depends upon whose ox is gored," which is to say, upon whose particular perspective we accept.

Indeed, psychologists recognize many meanings of the word "love." In addition to the Christian concept of unconditional, unselfish love, represented by the word "agape'," psychologists also recognize such categories as erotic love, companionate love and filial love. These categories of love fulfill quite different human needs.

As a verbal guide, the Bible cannot be free of such word problems. For example, the Beatitudes do not extol the "meek" as persons who lack courage, but as persons who learn, thus who are teachable. Also, modern scholars conclude that the sixth commandment admonishes us not to commit premeditated murder. It does not command us to refrain from killing when that is necessary, for example, to protect or to feed our families.

Then, of course, a meaning is determined by the particular arrangement of the groups of words. For example, consider a sign in a store window: "This store is closed because of the death of the owner temporarily." So, the particular arrangements of identical words are sometimes crucially important.

The linguistic problems are thus compounded for us if we try to read the Bible in a legalistic or strict dictionary sense of words. In a fervent attempt to get His message in the Bible across to us, God allowed metaphors and parables. A metaphor uses one word in the place of another in order to induce an analogy or comparison between them in an imaginative way. It says that, in some respect, they are the same. For example, God is a Father; God is a Son; God is a Holy Spirit. Jesus is a Shepherd.

A parable is a short fictitious narrative from which a moral or spiritual truth can be derived. Although the story itself is not true, it illustrates a message that is true. For example, the parable of the prodigal son tells us that the love and forgiveness of God is like the love and forgiveness of human fathers for their human sons. As the father of a son, I can have a good idea of the kind of love involved.

God says, "Be perfect." So, we must ask how we can be perfect. What behaviors define perfection? There are many other points in the Scriptures that give a more specific definition of perfection. For example, Paul said:

> Be imitators of God, therefore, as dearly loved children and live a life of love, just as Christ loved us and gave himself up for us as a fragrant offering and sacrifice to God.
>
> But among you there must not be even a hint of sexual immorality, or of any kind of impurity, or of greed, because these are improper for God's holy people. Nor should there be obscenity, foolish talk or coarse joking, which are out of place, but rather thanksgiving. For of this you can be sure: No immoral, impure or greedy person—such a man is an idolater—has any inheritance in the kingdom of Christ and of God. Let no one deceive you with empty words, for because of such things God's wrath comes on those who are disobedient. Therefore, do not be partners with them.
>
> For you were once darkness, but now you are light in the Lord. Live as children of light (for the fruit of the light consists in all goodness, righteousness and truth) and find out what pleases the Lord. Have nothing to do with fruitless deeds of darkness, but rather expose them. For it is shameful even to mention what the disobedient do in secret. But everything exposed by the light becomes visible, for it is light that makes everything visible. This is why it said:
>
> 'Wake up, O sleeper, rise from the dead, and Christ will shine on you.'[3]

For practical purposes, we must decide whether a particular proposed action would reflect "a hint of sexual immorality," or "obscenity" or "foolish talk." Obviously, we often have strong disagreements within the Christian, as well as secular, community about which behaviors satisfy those definitions. On more than one occasion, I have seen spiritually dedicated Christians walk out of church when the musical guests used rhythms on their guitars that have not been typically heard in church. I once knew a Christian who thought that drinking a cola beverage was surely immoral.

Some church members worry over the forms and trappings of worship in a spirit of combativeness and bad feelings. Therefore, the nominal issue may be trivial, but the spirit of argument is not. Jesus called this practice to be straining out a gnat while passing a camel.

You see, the problem is not that the Bible is inaccurate or false. The problem for us is that it requires us to read and to interpret it with the correct spirit. Thus, the Word in the Bible makes it difficult for us to live as we ought to live just by staying within the letter (wording) of some precisely worded laws. We are commanded to be perfect—not simply compliant with respect to some specific set of laws of our own making or interpretation.

I am certain that God is not concerned with the legal definitions drafted and recognized by our secular society. To be sure, a Christian will conscientiously obey secular laws that do not conflict with God's commandments. We must evaluate our behaviors according to the spirit of God's message in the Bible.

I can give two specific examples from my own experience. They both concern hit-and-run driving in an automobile. I witnessed the first case on a Sunday morning as my wife and I were on our way to church. An elderly lady drove out of a side street, through a red light, and very nearly hit the side of a car driven by a young girl. The girl avoided a collision by swerving her own car off the road and running into a fence. The lady never slowed down, although later events proved that she had been well aware of the accident. I dropped off my wife to help the girl, and then chased the lady in my automobile long enough to get her license number. The police later reported that *the lady had been on her way to church*. She did, in fact, attend a church service immediately after the accident, without having reported it.

The second story was reported to me by a reliable source soon after it happened. In this case, a lady accidentally drove her automobile into a building that, fortunately, was not occupied at the time. The building was substantially damaged. The lady then parked her car and completed an errand. She did not say a word about the accident to anyone, although she had easy access to a telephone. Then, she got in her car and drove off. When eyewitnesses later reported the event, those who knew her were surprised at her seemingly callous and surely illegal behavior. It seems that this lady was well known about town for her frequent pious utterings and religious posturings.

Apparently, having Christ on the tip of your tongue, or allegedly at your elbow while you are in church, is no guarantee that you will recognize your own personal sins in daily life, in or out of church. Surely, the ladies in the two stories above knew that their behaviors were clearly illegal. I wonder if they even considered that these behaviors were also sinful, and thus affronts to God?

Perhaps, these ladies did not understand the sinful nature of their acts because they were not aware of any specific commandment in the Bible that said, "Thou shalt not commit hit and run in thy automobile," or, "Thou shalt witness for Christ while driving thy automobile." But, surely, we could cite dozens of passages in the Bible that could cover the proper behavior in these situations very nicely.

Although you could hardly expect the Bible to mention an automobile, surely our behaviors while driving an automobile are covered by the teachings in the Bible. If nothing else, the wanton behavior is mean and unkind. Perhaps, too literal a reading of the Bible may even cause some people to lose God's message entirely.

Jesus often used metaphor, as I said. A good illustration occurs in the gospel of John when Jesus instructed Peter to feed His sheep. Because Jesus, as a carpenter, presumably did not possess any—or many—sheep, a literal reading of this passage makes little sense, or no sense at all. If, however, we understand that Jesus saw Himself as having a loving and caring relationship to His people, just as a shepherd has this same intimate relationship to his flock of sheep, the passage makes complete sense. And, in fact, it carries a most powerful instruction to all Christians to love and to care for their neighbors, who are surely loved by God, as the Good Shepherd.

Even the most literal interpreters of the Scriptures understand that Jesus was not talking specifically about the animals that graze. In any case, no one, to my knowledge, has taken Jesus so literally as to launch a global campaign, or to establish an organization, to feed all of the four-footed, wool-bearing animals on the planet.

Another example of Jesus' use of the parable was the story of the Good Samaritan. That parable gives Jesus' definition of a neighbor in an unambiguous way that is not possible with a simple dictionary definition. The story illustrates the meaning of the word "neighbor" in a powerful, meaningful and comprehensive way, necessarily understandable to everyone. Jesus leaves no legal loophole for us to escape our responsibilities to our neighbors.

Some of the greatest problems in interpreting the Scriptures come from applications to medicine, particularly the so-called right-to-life and death-with-dignity issues. Some dedicated Christians interpret the Bible to say that medical treatment attempts to thwart the will of God. Other Christians argue that heroic medical efforts to prolong life are actually necessary to fulfill the will of God. Surely, neither group would intentionally deny the omnipotence of God. I think that no one would ever actually say that giving medical treatment, or withholding it, could actually thwart the will of God. In my view, ordinarily God wills that His established laws of physics, biology and medicine be maintained. He does not cause a given person to become sick or to break a bone, or to be fatally injured, except in the sense that He established the laws that determine sicknesses, broken bones and fatal injuries, and He did not choose to suspend those laws in a particular instance. But, that is not the same as saying that God willed that particular sickness, broken bone or death to happen.

Therefore, it is not the fault of God's Word that some readers interpret it to forbid medical treatment entirely, while others argue that God wants feeding tubes and respirators to prolong the life of a brain-dead patient. These interpreters have left out the factor of love, and have gone straight to a particular set of their own rules. None of their actions or rules can control or suspend the functioning of the laws that God has established. All that anyone can do is to follow God's mandate to love, and try to convert that emotion of love into an act of love. Who can say without a context whether that act of love happens to be an aggressive medical intervention, or no intervention at all? The Bible must be interpreted prayerfully in order to translate it for guidance toward appropriate behaviors today.

Christian Witness

Fortunately, we do not have to rely entirely on our own personal interpretations of the Bible for guidance toward Christian living. We are aided by the interpretations of others in ways that are most important—namely, by what they do. Human models show what can actually be achieved in Christian living. In addition to the great men and women in history, there are family and friends that we have known directly and intimately to have achieved greatness of spirit in our world.

We know that no human being is perfect. But, the inevitable failures of the earthly saints merely prove that they were human, like us. They model correct behaviors for us in ways that are not likely to be misunderstood.

Unfortunately, we also have examples of un-Christian behaviors. Too many politicians and preachers in the electronic media have set false standards for us. In the words of Paul: "Some have wandered away from these [pure heart, good conscience, sincere faith] and turned to meaningless talk. They want to be teachers of the law, but they do not know what they are talking about or what they so confidently affirm" (bracketed material added).[4]

There are yet today those within the church, as well as outside of it, who serve as minions of the devil, who would confuse us by such practices as promoting false doctrines, providing false models of behavior, using meaningless talk and using their positions in the church for personal gain.[5] Therefore, we must use judgment in deciding which models to imitate, using all of our mental, emotional and spiritual powers.

The efforts of scoundrels can succeed only when we follow rules mindlessly. They fail to derail us when we keep our minds focused on following the will of God as we earnestly understand it. The false leaders must be strongly and steadfastly opposed. Jesus said so, and He was echoed by Paul. Unfortunately, the misguided souls are likely to make life very difficult for those dedicated Christians who oppose them.

My thoughts about evil distracters versus good models are summarized by a poem that I wrote a few years ago:

OH, GOD, WE KNOW

Oh, God, we know that some have said
There is no God, or Thou art dead,
Such doubters fail because they choose
To ply their search through sorry sloughs,
Of petty deals in murky blight,
Midst mindless men who shade Thy light.
But Thou art not in dreadful deeds,
Or tawdry thoughts from crooked creeds.

For Thou who holds Thyself from none
Hast proved it by Thy gift of Son,
Who trains our gaze, past hurt and smear,
On loving folk who witness here.
These human saints, tho' not divine,
Display a grace that mirrors Thine.
We glimpse thru them Thy greatest love,
Of One Who is, Who reigns above.

They seek no glory here below,
No cymbal clang, nor trumpet blow.
But every day their theme is heard;
Their light is spread through work and word.
With no pretense they deal with dross
That screens the glory of the cross.
So God we can Thy presence see,
When suff'ring servants model Thee.

The loaves and fishes that were shared,
Gave selfless sign that one boy cared.
And like a shepherd's constant care,
A parent's love is always there.
Thru these to us a path is giv'n,
An open way, a hint of heav'n.
Oh, God, we can Thy presence know
From suff'ring servants' lives below.

Thy power's in those who would Thy will,
Who suffer much, but praise Thee still.
So fill us with this strength and nerve,
With Job's resolve through all to serve.
Empow'r our faith to persevere,

And not be dulled by evil here.
Oh, God, may we Thy presence feel,
Thru suff'ring servants' waking zeal.

When saints display Thy great design,
I crave this Word, that It be mine.
My God, I want with them to stand,
And live my life as Thou command.
I raise my soul's affirming voice,
To tell the world I can rejoice.
For, God, I can Thy presence sing,
As suff'ring servant, hail Thee King!

Prayer/inspiration

God can inspire us with His truth. Such inspiration is more likely, I am sure, if we actively seek it. The primary avenue is through prayer, which necessarily involves such a search. I do not think that God is likely to inspire us with His message if we do not want it. That is why He gave us freedom to choose.

It is important for us to discriminate between types of prayer and non-prayer. Not every act that looks like prayer, or purports to be prayer, is in fact what prayer should be. I distinguish among three acts that relate to prayer: (1) True, or genuine, prayer; (2) Trivial prayer; and (3) Fake non-prayer.

True, or genuine, prayer is an interactive relationship with God. It is a serious personal conversation, a communication with God. Psychologists define communication as an intentional transmission of information about the world from one person to another. Because prayer involves a relationship, the communication travels in two directions: from man to God, and from God to man. Often we overlook the second part of the communication, and thus fail to listen to the communication from God. This attitude defeats a major purpose of prayer.

Why do we pray? We pray in order to make a connection with God, to bring ourselves closer to Him. It helps us to take on the mind of God, to achieve atonement. The process may take many forms: to worship; to give thanks; to confess; to ask for strength; to ask for guidance; to ask for comfort; to fulfill any Christian agenda.

When do we pray? Any time. You talk to significant others in your life whenever you desire interaction with them, especially to exchange information. Prayer requires no significant expenditure of time, because God knows your prayer even before you pray it. But, it may take a little time for you to understand your intentions, and to comprehend God's communication to you. In any case, prayer is a most efficient use of time, because atonement with God gives you the best basis for a good decision about the problems of life.

How do we pray? Jesus emphasized the importance of the right attitude for prayer. The prayer is worshipful and intercessory, emphasizing the dyadic connection. Group prayer is permissible as long as it does not lose this personal connection. Private prayer has the advantage of reduced distraction, and reduced temptation to pursue social agendas.

The term, "trivial prayer," may seem at first to be an oxymoron. Nevertheless, I call it prayer, because it is talking to God. But, it is not true prayer, because it is superficial and tries to be a one-way communication. It actually may be an insult to God, because it tends to take Him for granted. It tries to turn God into Santa Claus by presenting Him with a personal wish list. The stakes are trivial in the major scheme of things: "Let me score a touchdown; let me hit the jackpot; let me find my car keys."

The trivial prayer tries to turn God into a servant genie, sometimes eliminating the need for personal work and effort. The attitude is lazy. Indeed, the supplicant prefers a Godly miracle to personal achievement: "Let me pass the test without studying; let me know the proper grade for my students without the need to give and to score tests; let me diagnose the pathology without the bother of performing laboratory tests; let me pick the best investment without studying the records of the companies." I do not think that God is likely to provide for us that which He gave us the capability to provide for ourselves.

The fake non-prayer is not really a prayer, because the person is not talking to God. Jesus discussed this ploy when he told us in Matthew 6 how not to pray. For example, He said that we should not show off our supposed piety with acts to impress others. I would add that we should not recite mindlessly what we have memorized, because such is not conversation. And, we should not use our supposed prayer as a political ploy, to intimidate and to silence our opponents. The hypocrites claim—probably falsely—that God is on their side. This is a blasphemous use of the concept of prayer.

The fake non-prayer is a self-serving device that is unrelated to God. One is merely talking to one's self, or to a particular social group. Therefore, one cannot learn from it anything about God's will for us.

Frankly, at mealtime I often have to remind myself, while saying grace, to remember that I am praying to God. It is very easy just to slip into the recitation of a ritual. This is a real danger of all rituals.

Practical Feedback

There is positive practical feedback from Christian behaviors. We recite glibly such things as "Honesty is the best policy." But, do we really believe it? Although I do not believe in a strict version of the just-world hypothesis—that everyone always gets eventually what he or she deserves on this earth—I do believe that this principle is generally true. As discussed later in the book, I believe in what I call the "just-a-world hypothesis," which says that God established appropriate physical laws for His universe, and therefore behavior that is in harmony with those laws will generally have positive, beneficial consequences.

Sinful behaviors, those acts not in harmony with God's laws, will probably have harmful consequences. This does not mean that all of our troubles are caused by sin, but it does mean that our sin is likely to cause trouble for us in our lives on earth. But, nevertheless, adversity for a human is not always a direct punishment from God. Surely, we know not to repeat a behavior that, for us or others, leads to a poor result.

Reason

God gave us the ability to reason. Therefore, we can reasonably assume that He expects us to use it. When God's message seems to be contrary to reason, we have not been thinking effectively. For example, when we think that we perceive contradictions in the Scriptures, we have been interpreting them in too narrow or too literal a frame of reference.

Of course, we must do our best to ensure that we are following reason, and not simple personal desires. Unfortunately, there is no infallible technique for ensuring reason. The best advice, I think, it to consider prayerfully the possibility of a selfish motive.

The Armor of God

The Bible in Ephesians describes the full armor of God, thus describing the personal characteristics of a Christian:

> Therefore, put on the full armor of God, so that when the day of evil comes, you may be able to stand your ground, and after you have done everything, to stand. Stand firm then, with the belt of truth buckled around your waist, and with the breastplate of righteousness in place, and with your feet fitted with the readiness that comes from the gospel of peace. In addition, to all this, take up the shield of faith, with which you can extinguish all flaming arrows of the evil one. Take the helmet of salvation and the sword of the Spirit, which is the word of God.[6]

For today's society, I have proposed that we add to the armor a few pieces taken from modern psychology.[7] I have no doubt that all of these supplements are anticipated somewhere in the Scriptures.

Convert Love into Action

The first piece of supplemental armor is the ability to convert love into action. It is not sufficient simply to love without showing it in action. Indeed, one even questions the quality of a love that does not impel the person to helpful actions.

Tranquility

The next supplement to the armor is tranquility. The Christian must learn to relax, to quiet personal anguish. Only in this way can he or she be attentive enough to hear God's message, to make necessary discriminations and to make good choices. Psychologically, the person who is over-aroused from over-stimulation or personal worries is not able to make the good choices that are necessary to solve difficult ethical problems.

Sensitization

The third component of additional armor is sensitization, a responsiveness to human conditions everywhere. We must be sensitive to the problems of others, whether they are close neighbors or our more distant neighbors in other parts of the world.

Discrimination

Another piece of psychological armor, which is necessary in the modern world, is discrimination. In religious terms, this is called *discernment*. This is the ability to distinguish among different situations. I do not mean to propose situational ethics here. The truth of God is appropriate for all occasions; some things are absolutely right or wrong regardless of situations. But, nevertheless, some specific behaviors can be ethical or not depending upon the particular context. I personally put divorce and abortion in this category. I do not think that God disapproves of correcting mistakes, after the person has prayerfully and sensibly considered all alternatives.

Education

The next addition to modern Christian armor is education, meaning to bring out a person's potential for coping with life. The more we know about life, the better we can solve its problems. This knowledge does not replace our Christianity, because Christianity is a part of the necessary knowledge. We must not fear that our Christianity will fail to survive our intellectual scrutiny.

Evaluation

The next piece of modern psychological armor is the ability to evaluate. Evaluation means to process empirical evidence in order to reach a valid conclusion from that evidence. A proper evaluation cannot be made if one is biased. Even evidence which produces unpleasant conflicts with one's cherished ideas should not be ignored, or cavalierly dismissed.

Feeling Guilt

Next is the ability to feel guilt. The Christian must feel guilt when he or she has sinned. In Chapter 8, I discuss what I call a "glib confession of guilt." The word "glib" is an adjective meaning characterized by ease. Therefore, by this I mean that we are quick to confess in general terms that we are not perfect, and we similarly concede that others in the church are not perfect. But, we obstinately refuse to acknowledge particular sins. Therefore, there is no real pain of guilt, no sting of remorse. The harsh bite, and hence the true value, is gone because a non-specific confession is trite and easy. To be sure, a sincere confession should restore personal peace.

Compromise

The armor of compromise could be a weak spot in the Christian's armor as well. Discrimination is especially important here. Obviously, certain crucial basic principles must not be given up in efforts to reach compromise solutions. For example, the compromise must not involve basic personal integrity, or a departure from bedrock Christian beliefs. Under temptation in the wilderness, Jesus flatly rejected compromise. But, He also healed on the Sabbath, befriended a tax collector and spoke directly to a Samaritan woman.

Striving

Finally, the modern armor is augmented by the process of striving. The person must be motivated to hear, to learn, to choose, to achieve, etc. The motivation must be strong enough to withstand opposition. People who do not share the Christian's goals will naturally produce opposition. Therefore, there will always be opposition and strife for the person who tries to make improvements. The Christian must not fear stirring up controversy in a productive quest for truth and right.

Conclusion

God is flooding us with His message, in different ways, through different channels. To capture His message fully, we must use all of our human capacities. We must search for His word with our whole persons, not just emotionally, but also rationally and spiritually. When we have become sufficiently filled with His message, we will behave as He wishes us to behave.

The major problem in hearing God's message is that we, like the rich young ruler, would prefer to restrict His commandments to a short list of specific rules, which are relatively easier to follow. We foolishly think that such a list of formal rules for Christian behaviors will allow us to circumvent the basic instruction to be perfect. But, Christianity does not work that way. God is not naïve or foolish. And His central charges to us—love unconditionally, and be perfect—cannot be misinterpreted. God is quick to forgive us when we try and fail, but not, I think, if we deliberately misunderstand.

Although His word also reveals the highway to success in life on earth, that should not be our reason for accepting it. The Paradox of Christian Living tells us that a cynical pursuit of joy in life will make such joy unattainable. Joy is found only through loving outside of one's self, and thus living for others.

Notes

1. Holy Bible, New International Version (Grand Rapids, MI: Zondervan Publishing House, 1973), 1 Corinthians 13: 13.
2. E. Rae Harcum, *Biblical Guidance and Human Choices* (Williamsburg, VA: Cape Books, 1999).
3. Holy Bible, Ephesians 5: 1-14.
4. Holy Bible, 1 Timothy 1: 6-7.
5. E. Rae Harcum, *Saving Our Church: Five Systemic Diseases Pose a Vital Mission for the Organized Church* (Lanham, MD: Hamilton Books, 2009).
6. Holy Bible, Ephesians 6: 11-17.
7. Harcum, *Biblical Guidance*.

Chapter 5

Psychological Guidelines

This chapter continues the advice to Christians about how to improve themselves as Christians in order to be of greater help to their neighbors. To be sure, the proposed methods are educational, and not legal. Therefore, the following psychological guidelines for Christian living are not prescriptions, or rules, for particular behaviors to be performed in a Christian life. They are merely suggestions for appropriate personal characteristics to be adopted by a person who would witness and be a Christian mentor to other persons. Although these proposals flow directly from the results of psychological science, ultimately everything owes its being to God, as we are reassured in John: "Through him all things were made; without him nothing was made that has been made."[1]

The basic principles of guidance for effective daily living are therefore principles of Christian daily living. There is not the tiniest question in my mind that a Christian life is the best practical plan. Although Christian living may not work for us individually each time in the worldly sense of success, it does work in the sense of personal well-being. Even when there is a heavy personal cost for the individual, God's plan is still the most effective for a productive personal living and for a successful general society.

The present proposed guidelines for healthy living follow and expand the categories that I used some years ago.[2] As a mnemonic aid, these principles are listed under five rubrics, each beginning with the letter C: conviction, control, consistency, compassion and courage.

Conviction

A conviction is defined as a particularly strong belief in the validity of certain propositions and goals in life. Thus, a conviction is a core part of the person, a basic aspect of the individual human personality. A person with integrity necessarily acts on the basis of his or her convictions. In fact, without strong convictions, there can be no integrity.

The appearance of occasional disparities between a person's beliefs and his or her behaviors presents a significant problem for psychologists, because we ordinarily assume that there is a correspondence between beliefs and actions. Usually, the disparity is produced by the differential effects of other causal factors that are stronger than the beliefs. But, because convictions are especially strong beliefs, they are likely to prevail. Thus, a conviction provides a direction, a basis for guiding one's behaviors. On the basis of the belief in what is true, the person selects appropriate behaviors to achieve that truth.

In a religious context, we are likely to refer to these convictions as faith. Therefore, one has a faith to guide the way he or she lives. As psychologist Rollo May said, the major problem in life is that so many people do not have commitments to the things that give meaning to life.[3] A person without convictions is like a moving ship without a pilot or helmsman.

The conviction that one is attempting to do the will of God is therefore a prerequisite for using the remaining four of the C principles for successful Christian living. The most reliable basis for this conviction of truth and right is the sincere belief that one has succeeded in achieving beliefs that are at one with God. If a person is at one with God, his or her decisions will be effective in a practical sense. Therefore, a clear Christian conscience is the best measure of successful ethical living. Specifically, Christian living requires the conviction that some behaviors in given situations are simply wrong, because they are not consistent with the will of God.

The truly important truths to be gained from this book are in fact the ones that can be, and have been, incorporated into the readers' personal lives, made part of their personal consciences. Although one's religion must be personal, it must also be acted out in observable personal and professional relationships with others.

Christian living also means to eliminate sins of omission as well as sins of commission. Jesus strongly condemned the person with God-given talents who failed to use them.

These statements lead to the extremely important point that a deep conviction leads to a commitment to action, whatever the context. We can question the existence of an alleged conviction in a person when there is not an associated commitment by that person to act on the conviction. The commitment to action confirms the conviction. Success strengthens it.

The attempt to translate a conviction into specific acts helps us to clarify the precise nature of the conviction and its implications for Christian living. We must be clear about what we actually believe, if those beliefs are going to be the basis of our decisions and actions. Then, we can evaluate our actions in terms of the standards set by our beliefs.

Your own understanding of the truths in this book is crucial. Such understanding will undoubtedly be far more useful than any ideas or elaborations that I, or any other author, can supply. Valid meaning will spring from your own experiences, your own thinking. The specific propositions in this book should be merely food for your thought. Obviously, the various arguments in the book overlap, interact and support one another, because they are based on the universal model of our Christian beliefs.

Every choice in our lives is potentially a key event for our souls. This is true whether or not we understand our decisions in those terms. Often, we do not. Each decision inevitably moves us in a particular direction. Do we think about that final direction before we act? As Christians, we should make each decision in terms of its ultimate direction for us. Is the direction of our actions consistent with our convictions? Every decision has a consequence; it either affirms or denies Christ's everlasting love in the world. Our commission is to affirm it so that others may see it. We must ask ourselves: "Were my actions consistent with what I truly believe and openly profess?" Your sincere answer determines your level of integrity.

Control

Control means that the person will work actively toward the achievement of his or her personal goals, or a desired behavior in others. The control is not necessarily conscious. Indeed, we can choose behaviors automatically, without thinking. Probably, the automatic choices are most accurate reflections of our true motivations because we have not controlled them by deliberate thought of a self-serving sort. To be sure, life would be easier if we always did the right thing automatically, without conscious choice. But, such a happy state will not happen often. What we can do, and must do, is to strive for such a glorious condition where our deepest personal urges are to think of the welfare of others.

Control also means that we will not leave important decisions that affect us and our families to the discretion of others. For example, we should not leave it to someone else, professional or not, to make the decisions about the training and education of our children, religious or otherwise. I know from personal experience that professional educators advocated some horrendous decisions for my children. Only vigilance on our part was able to keep those plans out of our children's lives. This is not to assert that we should ignore the advice of professionals, or even knowledgeable non-professionals. It does mean that we should examine carefully and reflect on their recommendations before we take action. If we make the choice, we have the responsibility.

Because both my wife and I are professional social scientists and educators, we understand the difficulties in deciding on the best course of action for anyone with problems. Whenever we, as parents, yielded to persuasion against our own better judgment, we came to regret it. Do not give control to another human being to make a course of action that you really feel is unwise. This admonition is particularly important with respect to moral issues, especially those in the church.

Most of us do not have difficulty in agreeing that a person should control himself or herself. Some people, however, do not like the idea of one person controlling the behavior of others. The problem is primarily a semantic one, I think. The problem centers on the meaning of the word "control." We should not let some bad connotations of the word stop us from exercising such control.

As I have pointed out previously, psychologists use the word as a synonym for help, guidance, shaping and so forth.[4] Rarely is it used in the sense of forcing someone to do something against his or her will, unless that person for some reason does not have a competent personal will. Some persons, in fact, actually do not have competency to make reasonable choices. For example, we do not expect such competence from very young children, severely mentally retarded individuals or persons with disordered thinking. Indeed, we do not consider them capable of willfully committing crimes. So, they must be controlled by socialized, caring families and neighbors. Indeed, sometimes to control means to love.

It makes no sense to withhold help and guidance from someone because the giving of such help and guidance could be interpreted by someone else as unseemly interference in, or evil control over, the life of another. If the other person actually asked for help and guidance that you were capable of giving, any sin in this case would actually be in withholding the help.

The control over the behavior of another person can be established in many ways. Some of these methods are obvious and flagrant, and others are hidden and subtle. For example, it is possible to control by power and force. This is not always wrong. A parent might find it necessary to force a child to go to school or to church school, *if less forceful means have failed to be successful.*

More subtle controls are likely to be less stressful, and more effective in the long run. For example, help and guidance could be achieved by managing environmental conditions. The person could be kept away from cues in the environment that tended to elicit undesired behaviors; or such cues could be systematically eliminated from his or her environment. These harmful cues might be present in different crowds of people with whom the person came in frequent contact. Do not put another person, or yourself, in a situation that is likely to produce the cues that evoke undesired behaviors. Thus, a change of crowd, or role models, or environmental scenery, could be helpful.

Control over a person's behaviors could also be established by providing differential rewards for good behaviors. This is the most effective of management principles. This method entails the identification of good behaviors and finding ways to reward them. The rewards for good behavior are defined as any thing or situation that satisfies a need for the subject person. The guide or mentor discovers by a systematic process of trial and error what will reward a person who is not known to the guide. That is, the guide tries different possible rewards until he or she discovers what the subject person will work for in order to achieve that particular thing. To be sure, the parents tend to know from experience what their own child likes and what he or she dislikes. The parent who can control whether or not the child receives those rewards has virtually total power over the child. This procedure entails therefore an awesome responsibility, because such control of a person's rewards literally means to have virtually complete power to control the behavior of that person.

To be sure, the normal young child has a measure of freedom of will that must be considered. But, if the child's wishes are contrary to his or her best interests, the parent must make the decision about what the child is to do. Because the parents can control the rewards that the child will receive, the parents can control the child's behaviors. Be sure to develop the habit early! Do not wait until problems have developed. Do not let yourself, as a parent, for example, be tricked into thinking that the misbehavior of your very young child is merely cute, and not a problem. If you abdicate control when the child is young, do not expect to regain it—at least not easily—when the child becomes a teenager and the consequences of misbehavior become more serious.

A person's view of potential rewards can be changed. Therefore, what previously had been an incentive for motivating behavior may no longer be an incentive if it does not produce a rewarded behavior. It might even become a disincentive if it produces a behavior that is punished or associated with negative consequences. For example, the person's cognitive appraisal of an action could be changed by education. The behavior that had been condoned, and thus gained approval, could now be re-appraised by that person as harmful and sinful. For example, the bigoted person will become less bigoted when the society around him or her displays examples of love and brotherhood, and shows displeasure at behaviors that are disrespectful and harmful to other persons.

The identification of good behaviors means that the goals of the guide (i.e., coach, teacher, pastor, mentor, etc.) must be clearly defined so that a given behavior can be determined by the student to foster that goal or to hinder achievement of that goal. In general, the guide or mentor should never reward behaviors that do not lead to desired goals. For an obvious example, you do not reward the child for staying home from church school by letting him or her watch favorite television shows during the church-school hour.

This principle also means, of course, that you should not let yourself be rewarded for undesired behaviors. You yourself are not exempt from God's rules. Therefore, all readers are reminded that the same principles of control for other people can also be applied by us to ourselves to change our own particular behaviors. For example, we can control our exposure to tempting cues for poor behavior by simply choosing to be in another place, or by choosing a different group of people as friends or companions.

The issue of choosing the people with whom we will associate involves judgment in making the right decisions. Obviously, we cannot simply avoid outcasts and sinners. Jesus made that clear when He associated with the tax collector and the Samaritan woman at the well, and told the parable of the lost sheep. We cannot do His work adequately if we only preach to the converted. Therefore, we must show our Christian light to sinners. But, in so doing, we must be ever alert that they do not cause us to dim or diminish our own light. It is the direction of the influence and change that really matters. Are you strong enough to change the sinners, or actually vulnerable to their evil influences?

We can also improve our ability to make good decisions by controlling our emotions. For example, strong emotions, such as extreme fear and anger, can produce in us such a high level of arousal that we cannot perform certain functions at anywhere near our usual level of ability or control. We particularly experience a loss in our ability to make the discriminations that are necessary for intelligent and fair choices.

Psychological science tells us that the ability to control a situation reduces substantially the stress of that situation. Stress is an increase in unpleasant psychological arousal produced by input demands placed on a system which strains, or threatens to strain, its ability to function or to cope with the perceived threat. The reason for the psychological response of stress is that the person is not confident of his or her ability to cope with the threat. Therefore, the belief that he or she can cope constructively with the perceived threat, and thus control the situation, reduces or eliminates the perceived threat. The absence of stress is of course an important component of mental health.

The Bible is overflowing with assurances to the Christian that God will be with us to help us. Probably, our most familiar example is the Twenty-third Psalm: "Even though I walk through the valley of the shadow of death, I will fear no evil, for you are with me. Your rod and your staff, they comfort me."[5]

Consistency

Consistency in pursuing Christian goals is particularly important for one who would be a Christian role model. We cannot be consistent models of perfection, because no earthly model is perfect. But we can be consistent models of those who strive for perfection. Psychological science tells us that predictability of a situation, because of consistency, actually reduces the perceived stress of that situation. Judgments solidly based on convictions and conscience will necessarily be consistent.

The student-imitator must not be given mixed messages by inconsistent behaviors of the model. The inconsistency leads to confusion in the observer about what the model intends by his or her witnessing. It questions what standards the model truly represents. The meaning of the witness that is provided by the incorrect behaviors interferes with an understanding of what are the correct behaviors. The imitator of the model thus loses this basis for discriminating between correct and incorrect behaviors.

Although Christian ideals are applicable to any situation, job or personal perspective, judgment is required to know how to apply the principles to individual people and to particular situations. This is a real problem for the church. Just as intelligent people sometimes disagree on what is the wise action, committed Christians sometimes disagree about what is the Christian action in a specific situation. In such cases, there should be open discussion of the issues within the church, and even caring confrontation, if necessary. Whereas hidden agendas in the church are not Christian, open advocation for one's convictions is not only allowed by a Christian conscience, it is demanded by a Christian conscience.

Surely, we all have known people who seemed not to have personal convictions. They were consistent only in that they always followed the prevailing views of the people about them. Nevertheless, because different crowds often would entertain different views, their expressed views changed as often as the people about them. We often describe such people as "shallow," "arbitrary" and "trifling" because they have no depth of conviction, and thus are inconsistent in their actions. As we say, "They change with the wind."

The committed Christian consistently identifies, for example, some acts of hate as absolutely wrong despite the views of the crowd about him or her. Surely, the maintenance of consistent Christian convictions is far more valuable than the simple avoidance of conflict.

Some people try for consistency by drafting lists of formal rules to be followed. But, paradoxically, judgments based on rigid rules cannot be uniformly consistent. I believe firmly that fixed rules cannot be drafted to cover all changes or differences in situations that are bound to occur. For example, we even have had to make major amendments to the United States Constitution. Moreover, there are crucial substantive differences among the individuals to whom those rules allegedly apply.

There is also the problem of differences among individual persons in the interpretation of the rules. For example, let us consider potential dress codes for attendance at church services. Who would want to tackle the task of writing down a set of precise rules? When I was living in a tourist town, I was sometimes annoyed at the attire that I saw in church. I question the propriety of skimpy two-piece beach outfits on ladies in church on a Sunday. Some readers might say that God does not care about what we wear to church, as long as we are there. I would not argue with them. But, I do think that God cares about what is in our thoughts as we make choices of particular behaviors. For example, if a tourist had his or her luggage lost or stolen, I think that a loving and understanding God would not object to their sincere worship in whatever attire was available to them.

In any case, we need virtuous people who will at least try to make judgments based on Christian guidelines. We do not need dispassionate and disinterested people who will blindly enforce and follow rules based on personal whim or political correctness.

Compassion

Compassion is based on love, empathy and caring for other people. A person must be able to imagine himself or herself in the position of the other person, and have empathetic feelings accordingly. Modern life is complicated. Therefore, many of our decisions require choices from among many alternatives under stressful conditions. Under such conditions especially, we understand that we make mistakes, and therefore forgive ourselves.

Similarly, we understand that other people also make mistakes. In fact, psychologists never expect perfect performance from anyone, except on the very simplest of tasks. And, ethical judgments are often not simple to make. But, even with the very simple tasks, we often become preoccupied or distracted. We make mistakes especially under the extenuating circumstances of stressful conditions.

"Monday morning quarterbacking" is easy. A second-guessing of the players from the advantage of hindsight and oversight gains an advantage that the players on the field have not enjoyed. The stress is less when one has the immunity of spectator status, seated safely in the grandstand. The actor is trying to cope under conditions that he or she may not be able to control. What psychologists call "the actor-observer effect" is the tendency of a mere observer to attribute the failure of others (the actors) to the actors' own personal attributes and choices. But when we ourselves are the actors, we tend to attribute our own failures to certain exigencies in the environment that are perceived as beyond our control. Thus, the need for compassion for anyone under his or her particular circumstances is rather obvious.

Christians should agree also that the need for compassion for one's own self is equally important. Why should Christians not give themselves the benefit of the same compassion that they would willingly accord to others? This message should not be taken to give a license for Christians to forego active consciences. It does mean, however, that Christians should not burden themselves with unreasonable guilt. Just as God forgives us when we repent, we must likewise forgive ourselves when we repent.

Courage

Knowing which is the Christian behavior to make in a given situation is of little value when one does not have the necessary motivation to produce that behavior. Indeed, often it is necessary to have real courage to make decisions that are unpopular. Going against the crowd is always aversive to us. Psychologists recognize the strong push toward making responses that conform to our perception of the usual behaviors of the people around us. We want to be part of the group, and we feel uncomfortable whenever we are made to feel different from the rest of the group.

Failure to conform to the norms of the group may even entail unpleasant consequences. Frequently, there are newspaper accounts of the harsh treatments given to the "whistle-blowers" who have called attention of the authorities to immoral or illegal practices of their bosses, co-workers or colleagues. In fact, the social penalties inflicted on the informants may actually be more severe than the legal punishments meted out to the perpetrators of the wrongful acts. For example, the non-conformist may be "silenced," "shunned" or otherwise ostracized from full membership or participation in the group.

The Christian who is trying to live the Christian life is bound to run into opposition. This truth applies even to activities within the church, as well as to secular situations. Just as individual Christians are not perfect, church organizations of people are not perfect either. The Christian needs not only the wisdom to detect flaws in the organization, but the courage to report those imperfections to the persons who can correct them.

Courage is required because often caring confrontation is viewed by others as simply criticism, interference and aggression. The Christian needs the courage to persevere in the face of opposition that may even become abusive and physical. Even those calling for reforms within the church can be victims of such abuse and retaliation from the members who see themselves as injured. In fact, the sociologist, Enroth, described some churches and church leaders who literally became abusive, physically and mentally, to dissident members within their congregations.[6]

Paul warned Christians about the dangers of creating dissention in the church. He considered that some false issues, concerning such as the practice of circumcision and other such rituals, were inconsequential and distracting to the main goals of the Christian. Paul counseled opposition to those persons who tried to inject such false issues into the discussion of Christian beliefs. The true issue is whether it is the ritual or the spirit that is essential to a Christian.

One also needs courage in order to persevere in spite of personal failures and disappointments. Striving for personal perfection will surely lead to the perception of many personal failures. This is a somewhat different kind of courage. For example, repeated failures to make changes in a given life situation may give rise to a "what's-the-use?" attitude. Psychologists refer to this psychological state as "learned helplessness."[7] It is especially harmful because it generalizes to other problem situations as well. The defeated person just gives up altogether, even on easier tasks.

This situation is particularly hurtful if the individual rejection is associated with personal animosity from those who are in need of correction. But Jesus said, "Follow me." He did not say, "Follow me, providing there is earthly reward in it, and no aversive consequences."

Conclusion

Attempts to live a Christian life must be guided by the degree of personal closeness to God rather than by rigid rules. You cannot rely on someone else to tell you, or to draft a rule to tell you, what are the Christian responses in all situations that you are likely to face. And, the neighbor who might "know" the correct answer is not likely to be present when you need him or her. So, you probably will be forced to rely on your own conscience. Therefore, you must develop your own criteria for Christian living.

The danger in proposing general guidelines for ethical living, such as I have done, is that the reader comes to view these suggestions for adopting Christian behaviors as rules themselves. For example, consistency does not imply that the person invariably makes the same response despite critical changes in situations and circumstances. Indeed, two situations are never exactly the same. For example, the principle of compassion may indicate that some loosening of the standards for consistency is appropriate.

In summary, no set of suggestions, guidelines or rules should cause a committed Christian to make a response that he or she clearly considers to be inappropriate, foolish or sinful under the circumstances. The Great Commandment is the unwavering standard. But, for specific applications, it must be interpreted according to a committed Christian conscience.

Notes

1. Holy Bible, New International Version (Grand Rapids, MI: Zondervan Publishing House, 1973), John 1: 3
2. E. Rae Harcum, *Psychology for Daily Living* (Chicago: Nelson-Hall, 1979).
3. Rollo May, in M. H. Hall, An Interview with "Mr. Humanist," Rollo May, *Psychology Today,* 1, 24-29, 72-73, 26.
4. Harcum, *Psychology for Daily Living.*
5. Holy Bible, Psalm 23: 4.
6. Ronald M. Enroth, *Churches That Abuse* (Grand Rapids, MI: Zondervan Publishing House, 1992).
7. M. E. P. Seligman, Learned helplessness, in *Depression: Concepts, Controversies, and Some New Facts*, ed. J. Levitt, B. Rubin, & J. Brooks (Hillsdale, NJ: Erlbaum Publishers, 1983).

Chapter 6

Conditional Forgiveness

This chapter on forgiveness has been particularly difficult for me to write because my ideas on the subject are so different from those that I have heard so often from the pulpit. I do not claim to be an expert on forgiveness. Nevertheless, it is a problem that we all must solve, if we are to have mental health and the peace that goes with it. In fact, mental health professionals have come to value the role of forgiveness in psychotherapy.[1] Hartz points out that the goal is to free the patient of anger over past offenses.[2] He includes self-forgiveness in this assessment, as well as forgiveness of others.

I am totally confident on one point, made clearly in the Bible: If your neighbor repents, you surely must forgive, immediately and without reservation. I am less confident of the second point, that gracious forgiveness is not necessary, and perhaps not even a good thing, if your neighbor refuses to repent.

One of my greatest problems as a Christian comes from having to deal with persons who have harmed me and later failed to show remorse. Some Christians offer as a simple solution for this problem that one is to forgive unconditionally because you love. But, I do not think that Jesus advocated and modeled universal, immediate, unconditional forgiveness in all instances, despite His final act on the cross. Two examples of Jesus withholding forgiveness, at least temporarily, come to mind. The first was when Jesus berated the Pharisees for being liars and hypocrites, and the second was the scourging of the moneychangers in the synagogue.

Problems of Forgiveness

The first problem concerning forgiveness is whether or not to forgive. I have often heard it said from the pulpit that Jesus' plea from the cross for forgiveness of His persecutors was a model to us for immediate, total and unconditional forgiveness. But, Jesus did add a condition to the forgiveness that He requested: "for they do not know what they are doing."[3]

Certainly, a sin against us is less severe, and easier to forgive, if it is committed in ignorance, rather than knowingly and deliberately. Nevertheless, I do think that failure to forgive is most often our sin that makes us different from Jesus.

The problem with forgiveness begins with the actual meaning of the word. The word has an absolute quality such that it would appear that you either forgive or you do not. But, it seems that the actual situations are often too complex to permit such an either/or decision. Perhaps, a degree of forgiveness, or a conditional forgiveness, is possible.

One point is nevertheless abundantly clear, as I have said: you must forgive, presumably completely, if the sinner repents and sincerely asks for forgiveness. As Luke said: "So watch yourselves. If your brother sins, rebuke him, and if he repents, forgive him. If he sins against you seven times in a day, and seven times comes back to you and says, 'I repent,' forgive him."[4]

You gain nothing spiritually or psychologically, and add nothing to the spiritual growth of others, if the sinner repents and you decline to forgive. The value of the rebuke and the repentance process has already been achieved. Under such a circumstance, the failure to forgive models meanness, and not the Christian spirit of love.

When the person who has offended freely acknowledges that fact and sincerely asks for forgiveness, the Christian response thus is easy to know. Understanding that everyone makes mistakes, we can willingly extend forgiveness. Like the father in the parable of the prodigal son, we can forgive simply because the prodigal asks for forgiveness, and we love him or her.

But, the above passage from Luke does not speak to the question of possible forgiveness if the offender does *not* repent. Thus, in the absence of such repentance, the offended person is apparently allowed the judgment to forgive or not. Therefore, when the person offends and harms us, and refuses to repent, even after confrontation, I think that the Bible does not mandate an immediate and unconditional forgiveness.

The absolutely crucial question at this point is whether or not it is possible to love, but not to forgive. My partial answer to this question depends upon the depth of love, and the level of forgiveness. Love can be so deep that it blinds us to reality, and that is not always good. Forgiveness can be so complete that it entails forgetting as well, and that is not always good. For example, you can forgive someone for not repaying a debt to you, but you may not wish to lend money to that person again. I do not think that being Christian forces us to be stupid on psychological questions. We can forget the resentment and bad feelings without forgetting the event.

A second problem of forgiveness concerns when to give it. A delay in forgiving can allow time for an offender to reflect on his or her offense, and thus repent. Forgiveness that is too quick essentially removes the full consequences of the offense.

God's Way

The Bible surely does not condone the human desire for revenge. When an offense is committed without any sign of contrition, we have problems with forgiving the offender, because we want justice. Our human logic says, "What goes around, comes around." But, often we want a just world simply so that our enemies will eventually get what they deserve.

That is the human way. But, it surely is not God's way. Jesus instructed us otherwise in the Sermon on the Mount:

> Ye have heard that it hath been said, An eye for an eye, and a tooth for a tooth: But I say unto you, That ye resist not evil; but whosoever shall smite thee on thy right cheek, turn to him the other also. And if any man will sue thee at the law, and take away thy coat, let him have thy cloak also. And whosoever shall compel thee to go a mile, go with him twain. Give to him that asketh thee, and from him that would borrow of thee turn not thou away. Ye have heard that it hath been said, Thou shalt love thy neighbor, and hate thine enemy: But I say unto you, Love your enemies, bless them that curse you, do good to them that hate you, and pray for them which despitefully use you, and persecute you; That ye may be the children of your Father which is in heaven: for he maketh his sun to rise on the evil and on the good, and sendeth rain on the just and on the unjust. For if ye love them which love you, what reward have ye? Do not even the publicans the same? And if ye salute your brethren only, what do ye more than others? Do not even the publicans the same? Be ye therefore perfect, even as your Father which is in heaven is perfect.[5]

Some of these instructions thoroughly shock us if we evaluate them out of context. For example, we are literally told in this passage not to resist evil. Then, we think that combating evil is exactly what Christian soldiers are expected to do. But, the rest of the passage provides the proper context. In one of the most familiar passages in the Bible, Jesus tells through parable the relation between God and man with respect to forgiveness, as follows:

> Then Peter came to Jesus and asked, 'Lord, how many times shall I forgive my brother when he sins against me? Up to seven times?'
> Jesus answered, "I tell you, not seven times, but seventy-seven times.
> Therefore, the kingdom of heaven is like a king who wanted to settle accounts with his servants. As he began the settlement, a man who owed him ten thousand talents was brought to him. Since he was not able to pay, the master ordered that he and his wife and his children and all that he had be sold to repay the debt.
> The servant fell on his knees before him. 'Be patient with me,' he begged, 'and I will pay back everything.' The servant's master took pity on him, canceled the debt and let him go.
> But when that servant went out, he found one of his fellow servants who owed him a hundred denarii. He grabbed him and began to choke him. 'Pay back what you owe me!' he demanded.
> His fellow servant fell to his knees and begged him, 'Be patient with me, and I will pay you back.'
> But he refused. Instead, he went off and had the man thrown into prison until he could pay the debt. When the other servants saw what had happened, they were greatly distressed and went and told their master everything that had happened.
> Then the master called the servant in. 'You wicked servant,' he said,

> 'I canceled all that debt of yours because you begged me to. Shouldn't you have had mercy on your fellow servant just as I had on you?' In anger his master turned him over to the jailers until he could pay back all he owed.
> This is how my heavenly Father will treat each of you unless you forgive your brother from your heart.[6]

I note three messages in this passage. First, Jesus is referring to evils against you as a person. He was not referring to evils performed against the work and the people of the Lord that could be prevented or stopped by your active opposition.

Second, I think that Jesus was objecting to a fixed rule for establishing the number of turnings of the cheek that were required. He was not establishing a new rule that required unlimited turnings of the cheek.

Third, Jesus asserted that God does not always forgive, or that there are some things that God does not forgive. He said that God will not forgive those who refuse to forgive others. Therefore, because God Himself does not forgive under some circumstances, presumably there are circumstances in which we are not required to forgive.

But, there is a complication in the interpretation of Jesus' parable: His parable refers specifically to debts having cash equivalents, rather than to personal efforts or injuries, or affronts to God and the church. To owe someone money seems categorically different from committing a sin against that person, or breaking Gods' law. Surely, a person cannot repent from owing you money, unless he or she was able to pay the debt, and then deliberately refused to pay it. Presumably, Jesus did not have in mind a situation in which the servant was able to pay, or was unwilling to pay if given time for repayment. Therefore, the servant was caught in a circumstance beyond his or her control, and did not have the choice to repay immediately. But, that servant did have a choice about canceling the debt that another owed him. Because he did not, his master reconsidered his earlier decision, and held his servant accountable for the large debt. Therefore, there had been some implied limitation or restriction on the master's earlier forgiveness. He obviously had not forgotten the episode. His earlier forgiveness was therefore probationary. But, is that possible? It is rather sobering to think that God will rescind earlier forgiveness, if we sin again.

If Jesus had meant that we should forgive endlessly, why did the master in the parable not forgive his servant for demanding repayment of the debt owed to him? My answer is that the master was genuine in the initial forgiveness, but had a reasonable basis for withholding his forgiveness in the second case.

Jesus was very clear that God will treat us the same way. Therefore, Jesus shows us a model of a God who judges that some deliberate sins are not to be forgiven, at least not immediately. God may choose to rebuke or punish us before He forgives us.

But, suppose in Jesus' parable the servant had been able to pay his master, and had refused. Would the master have forgiven the debt in the first place? I am not sure that he would have, just as I am not sure that God will forgive us if we deliberately refuse to pay our debts. If we have a choice, and deliberately make the wrong one, I think that He will hold us accountable until we make the right choice.

I think that our reasonable God understands and appreciates differences in situations. He does not hold us accountable for actions beyond our personal control, just as in theory our society does not hold us responsible for behaviors that we could not help. Even when we make bad choices, there can be mitigating or extenuating circumstances that indicate that mercy is appropriate, and He is surely merciful.

The situation is different when we deliberately commit sins against God, or our fellow human beings. If we intentionally make the bad choices, when we could have done otherwise, God's grace is not immediate and automatic, I think. For example, I understand the Bible to say that God does not overlook or forgive open rebellion against His authority. In Exodus 23:21 and in Joshua 24:19, the people of Israel are admonished that God would not forgive their rebellion and sins against Him. Jesus Himself said explicitly in Matthew "For if you forgive men when they sin against you, your heavenly Father will also forgive you. But if you do not forgive men their sins, your Father will not forgive your sins."[7] That statement seems to me to be rather unambiguous. It seems right, and consistent with my understanding of a loving, but sensible, God.

This also seems to be Jesus' understanding of God's stance on forgiveness. He said, in Luke: "Do not judge, and you will not be judged. Do not condemn, and you will not be condemned. Forgive, and you will be forgiven."[8] And again in Luke, He said: "So watch yourselves. If your brother sins, rebuke him, and if he repents, forgive him. If he sins against you seven times in a day, and seven times comes back to you and says, 'I repent,' forgive him."[9]

Jesus said that, if you forgive men their sins, God will forgive you. I do not like to play word games with passages in the Bible, but at this point an examination of the word "if" can be helpful. It introduces a condition or supposition by saying, "in the event that," and "on condition that." Therefore, the condition must be met before the conditional event will happen. So, it is clear that God will forgive you *if* you repent and forgive others when they repent. It is also clear that God expects and requires you to forgive someone if he or she repents and forgives. Again, it is not required of you to forgive if the offender does not repent or forgive.

Therefore, God loves unconditionally, but He also has rules which He follows with integrity. Therefore, we should not presume God's grace if we are unrepentant and unforgiving. Because He is perfect, we too should not allow others to presume our forgiveness if they are unrepentant and unforgiving. We can assume God's grace, but we cannot presume it if we are rebellious. Accordingly, those we love can assume our forgiveness, but they cannot presume it if they have not forgiven others or been repentant.

To be sure, it may seem strange to suggest that Jesus did not instantaneously and unconditionally forgive sinners. His sublime act of forgiveness on the cross is often cited as proof to the contrary, as I said. But, although Jesus, on the cross, displayed the ultimate act of forgiveness, it was in fact conditional. He knew that they needed forgiveness, because they chose to crucify Him. But, He also knew that their choice of the action was not fully informed, thus providing a mitigating circumstance. We are left to speculate about what Jesus would have done if His executioners had understood who He was, and had deliberately and unrepentantly proceeded with the execution. Because God and Jesus love unconditionally, but forgive conditionally, it is possible to love and not forgive. I have a very difficult time in trying to understand how that could work, because of the emotional change that is involved in forgiveness. In forgiveness, one does not simply give up the hope or need for revenge or compensation, but also the emotions of resentment and alienation. In a word, some level of love is restored.

I think that we must look to psychology to resolve this mystery. We cannot induce people to change their ways of behaving for the better if their poor behaviors do not have adverse consequences. If people felt that all of their transgressions were immediately forgiven, there would be no practical point in distinguishing between good and bad behaviors. True repentance would become far more difficult to achieve. The perfect response of the offended person would be more likely to turn the transgressor toward the Lord, and to hasten the advent of God's Kingdom on earth.

The person who has sinned against you will also not be caused by your resistance to mend his or her ways. In fact, your resistance during and after the act can be perceived to verify and justify the original offense against you. Turning the cheek and loving your tormentor will witness to the Word of the Lord in a most positive and powerful way. I might add parenthetically that such Christian actions will probably be more effective in stopping the abuse than any kind of hostile resistance that you might offer. Therefore, I strongly believe that Christian witnessing is the most effective approach to successful living in this world. Of course, turning the cheek and offering forgiveness are not the same. One is an overt behavior, which may or may not reflect forgiveness, which is a feeling in the soul. That was the point that Jesus made in rebuking Peter for setting a limit on the number of times that he would turn the cheek. The act should witness love and forbearance, not ignorance of the psychology of interpersonal relations. I think that Jesus' message is that the Christian cannot arbitrarily choose beforehand the number of turnings that establish a limit of love, and the degree to which further sin by the transgressor should be encouraged by inaction.

At this point, I am borrowing the psychological reasoning of a particular practical plan for dealing with problem children. The plan, called Tough Love, entails a confrontation and a setting of limits on those behaviors that will be tolerated. I should emphasize that the limitations are on undesired behaviors, and not on love for the problem child. The child is supported when he or she produces desired behaviors, and definitely not protected from the consequences of undesired behaviors.

This approach corresponds with Christian teachings. We should note that in 2 Timothy, Paul advised Timothy to rebuke and to encourage.[10] Psychologically, encouragement does not necessarily imply forgiveness. Unconditional, blanket forgiveness may only encourage the original sinful behaviors. This interpretation is further supported by Paul's later words in the message to Timothy: "But you, keep your head in all situations, endure hardship, do the work of an evangelist . . ."[11] You see, forgiveness is good for the peace of mind of the offended person, but it may not help to bring the sinner to the Lord. Therefore, the best course is for the Christian to forgive in his or her heart and soul, and to show love for the transgressor, but not necessarily to communicate overtly forgiveness to the transgressor. This type of tough love may be necessary to help the sinner turn his or her life around.

Psychotherapists emphasize this essential training in reality. The child must understand that the nature of things is that actions beget consequences. The child must be protected from danger, but not from an understanding that his or her poor behaviors can have adverse consequences for him or her as an individual. This may even entail appropriate punishment for bad behavior. But, the purpose should be teaching, not revenge.

To know the right path and to walk the path of forgiveness are not the same, of course. Unfortunately, too often I know what I should do, but I cannot bring myself to do it. Even the apostle Paul had this problem. So, it is a human frailty. The failure to love and to forgive adds burdens to our minds and souls. These human failures are understandable in some cases. For example, how can I forgive the bombers of the federal building in Oklahoma City? How can I forgive those who every night commit cold-blooded murder on the streets of our cities? How can I love and forgive someone who falsely and deliberately says bad things about one of my loved ones, without remorse? The memory is written on my mind with indelible mental ink.

How can I forget the hurtful letter from the rejected applicant for a license as a psychologist in the state of Virginia when I was chairman of the state licensing board? In writing, available to the public, he called me unfair and a liar when our board refused to grant him a license. I felt genuine pain every time we had to reject a candidate for licensure. All of us on the board were making great personal sacrifices to serve and protect the people of the Commonwealth of Virginia, even to accepting the viable risk of civil lawsuits that could literally impoverish our families. A favorite tactic of rejected applicants was to have our lawyers remind us that we could be sued for punitive damages that could wipe out every penny of our personal wealth. Imagine the reluctance that I felt in asking my wife to accept such a real risk! I was thus distressed to be hostilely confronted with this evidence that my work was not appreciated, and even my personal character was callously impugned.

Unquestionably, it was my professional, civic and Christian duty to resist this man in his pursuit of a license. So, my sin was not in resisting this man. Surely, it was not wrong to promote conflict with him by my lawful actions. My sin was my failure to love this man.

All of my colleagues on the board strongly advised me to forget it, to consider the source. They said that anyone who knew me would not pay any attention to the man's charges. The man was obviously trying to manipulate me and the system to get what he wanted. Intellectually, I understood that very well. My reaction was not rational, but emotional. I was ready to resign from the board, despite the protests of my fellow board members. I thought and prayed about the situation almost continuously for many days, but to no avail.

Then, by what I can only call a miracle, suddenly my whole perspective on the conflict drastically changed. One day, I simply realized that the man's artful and mean allegations did not matter to me any more. Whereas I had been absolutely unable to feel relief by my own efforts, I now could accept emotionally what my intellect had understood long before. Thus, I had first-person knowledge of the healing power of God. What I could not do by my best personal striving, He gave as a gift.

Maybe, someday God will similarly lift the grudge that I hold against this man. I have tried to love and forgive. But, I know that truly, deep down, I have not. I know that I have not, because there really is no peace there, even though now I cannot even remember the man's name. To be sure, after all of these years, I do not often think about this man. But, when I do, there is no peace. I am sure that my continued resentment would not bother that man. To my knowledge, he has never repented. My failure to forgive thus punishes only me, blocking my psychological peace, in a way that his false allegations never could. I will know when I have been successful, because then I will be able to think about the man with peace in my soul.

Practical Value

Forgiveness not only opens the door to reconciliation to others, and to God, but it also has, as I said, a psychotherapeutic effect on the person who forgives. Forgiveness has become a useful tool in psychotherapy by professionals in helping the patient to reduce his or her anger. The process includes self-forgiveness as well as forgiveness for the offenses of others. The person who forgives gives up the resentments that can be destructive to personal mental health. McCullough, Bono and Root concluded that, "Given the empirically established links between religiousness and forgiveness, and their independent association with measures of health and well-being, it seems plausible that some of the beneficial influences of religion on health and well-being occurs because religion encourages people to practice forgiveness in their relationships with friends and family."[12] These authors caution, however, that important research relating these three concepts in a causal way have not been done.

So, my belief is that, as a Christian, I should actively oppose the perpetrators of evil, if I can prevent or stop their evil acts. But, retaliation and resentment against them after the fact is not Christian. Instead, we must try to love them and to rehabilitate them. Nevertheless, we must take whatever steps are necessary to prevent them from doing evil in the future.

William Booth, a Baptist minister, makes this point very well in the context of leaders who fail us.[13] A rush to forgiveness tends to belittle the sin, and also to pre-empt active redemption. The offender is not confronted and rebuked, and therefore he or she is not given the opportunity to come forward with repentance. And without repentance, as Booth says, there can be no reconciliation. There must be some pain in the full realization and confession of guilt by the perpetrator for the process to move forward to a better relationship to God and the offended neighbors.

This operation makes sense psychologically as well as spiritually. The very process of psychotherapy is painful as the person confronts and attempts to deal with his or her harmful behaviors and beliefs. The personal effort and sense of responsibility are essential. As Mahoney, a psychologist, said:

> I have never "cured" a client of a mental disease; I do not know what that would be like. But I have seen people transcend and transform painful constraints on their personal freedom, and the experience has been both humbling and inspiring.[14]

Therefore, the rehabilitation process is not likely to be instantaneous. The person needs time to work through his or her problems with the aid of the psychotherapist. Similarly, the Christian counselor or friend may help, but the offender must work through to a personal realization of guilt and the need to repent.

A global act of unspecified repentance will not work, because the problem—the sin—has not been identified. Although we blithely acknowledge ourselves as sinners, as we do in the Lord's Prayer, and routinely offer corporate prayers for the forgiveness of our sins each Sunday, often we do not specifically identify the sins. Therefore, these prayers are often what I call "glib confessions" of "trite guilt." Through these alleged confessions, we neatly evade the entire issue of repentance.

Repentance for such unspecified sins is really not repentance at all. Booth made this point in reference to the head of a national organization who had been charged with mishandling funds of the organization.[15] The official had requested forgiveness for "unspecified 'tremendous mistakes.'" Booth's point is that the failure to be specific in the supposed apology and statement of repentance revealed that the proper spirit of contrition was not present. Therefore, the sinner is not motivated to change himself or herself, and reconciliation is impossible. True reconciliation must be mutual; it cannot be accorded in a unilateral act of forgiveness, no matter how loving, or well-meaning, the act itself.

Another factor in our decision about overt acts of forgiveness is the degree to which the person was responsible for his or her wrongful behaviors. Our society ordinarily holds the person responsible only for those behaviors that are freely chosen. In other words, psychologists have found that we blame a person for his or her bad behaviors only when we consider that it was in his or her power to behave otherwise. If a behavior was beyond the control of the person's will to control it, then the person actually merits understanding, rather than forgiveness. In fact, the act of understanding is a kind of forgiveness. This is what I think that Jesus meant on the cross when He asked the Father to forgive His executioners. They were mindless victims of their inherited human nature and the bloodthirsty culture.

Regardless of our decisions about forgiveness, we should not assume that forgiveness implies forgetfulness. As Booth pointed out, each sin takes its toll.[16] You cannot un-ring a bell. Actually, the ultimate choice of the appropriate behavior is based more on psychological factors, rather than spiritual issues. The most positive thing to say is that we should all learn from experience. God gave us a brain that allows us to profit from experience. To have paid for a crime, or to be pardoned for it, does not mean that everyone should trust that person in the future. Forgiveness for sin does not remove the need for re-establishing a new, clean record for trustworthiness.

Summary

Reconciliation to God is always possible for us. The apostle Paul achieved it. We still do not know the nature of his thorn in the flesh. And Paul started out a lot farther away from reconciliation than most of us.

We are not terribly evil. We are not like the prodigal son who became estranged from God through riotous living. We are more like the older brother, a good son and responsible citizen. He was the one, however, who could not even forgive his remorseful brother, or his father, who begged for it. So, in the end, the older brother was actually the sinful son. We must want reconciliation with God so much that we are willing to try to become reconciled with all of our neighbors, even those who do not deserve it. Then God will be reconciled with us, even though we do not deserve it.

Notes

1. Gary W. Hartz, *Spirituality and Mental Health: Clinical Applications* (Binghamton, NY: The Haworth Press, 2009). Michael E. McCullough, Giacomo Bono and Lindsey M. Root, Religion and Forgiveness. In *Handbook of the Psychology of Religion and Spirituality*, eds. Raymond F. Paloutzian and Crystal L. Park (New York: The Guilford Press, 2005), 394-411.
2. Hartz. *Spirituality and Mental Health.*
3. Holy Bible, New International Version (Grand Rapids, MI: Zondervan Publishing House, 1973), Luke 23:34.
4. Holy Bible, Luke 17: 3-4.
5. Holy Bible, Matthew 6: 38-48.
6. Holy Bible, Matthew 18: 21-35.
7. Holy Bible, Matthew 6: 14-15.
8. Holy Bible, Luke 6: 37.
9. Holy Bible, Luke 16: 3-4.
10. Holy Bible, 2 Timothy 4: 2.
11. Holy Bible, 2 Timothy 4: 4-5
12. McCullough, Bono and Root, *Religion and Forgiveness*, 406.
13. William Booth, Forgiveness may not lead to real reconciliation. *Daily Press*, Newport News, VA, September 22, 1997, D7.
14. Michael J. Mahoney, Psychology and human change processes. In *Cognition and Psychotherapy*, eds. Michael J. Mahoney and A. Freeman (New York: Plenum Press, 1985), 3-48.
15. Booth, Forgiveness may not lead to real conciliation, D7.
16. *ibid.*

PART III. GOD'S GIFT OF CHOICE

Chapter 7

Empowered Decisions

As a psychologist, I have adopted and promulgated the Humanistic theoretical position that human beings have the capacity to make choices of behaviors.[1] This psychological theory is entirely consistent with Christian theology.[2] Because human beings have the God-given capacity to choose, it follows that we have the responsibility to choose wisely. The Bible is very clear on this point in the Psalms, as follows:

> Do not be like the horse or the mule, which have no understanding but must be controlled by bit and bridle or they will not come to you. Many are the woes of the wicked, but the Lord's unfailing love surrounds the man who trusts in him. Rejoice in the Lord and be glad, you righteous; sing, all you who are upright in heart![3]

Joshua emphasized to the people of Israel that they had to make personal choices to serve either the Lord, or to serve false gods. This issue of personal choice is a frequent theme throughout the Bible. Joshua emphasized also that we are judged by the choices, as follows:

> Now fear the Lord and serve him with all faithfulness. Throw away the gods your forefathers worshiped beyond the River and in Egypt, and serve the Lord. But if serving the Lord seems undesirable to you, then choose for yourselves this day whom you will serve, whether the gods your forefathers served beyond the River, or the gods of the Amorites, in whose land you are living. But as for me and my household, we will serve the Lord.[4]

Paul also made it clear in his letter to the Galatians that human beings are free to choose a spiritual life or a life of sin: "You, my brothers, were called to be free. But do not use your freedom to indulge the sinful nature; rather, serve one another in love."[5] Thus, to choose to serve the Lord is to choose to serve His people. The one choice controls the other. In fact, Christians believe that people are Christian or non-Christian for the very reason that their beliefs as persons cause them to choose Christian behaviors over non-Christian acts.

Unfortunately, the views of psychology that have most often been presented in the popular books and in the modern media have been incompatible with this most basic of Christian tenets. For example, both the Psychoanalytic school of thought, fathered by Sigmund Freud[6] ,and the Behavioristic school of thought, championed by B. F. Skinner[7], have denied the ability of human beings to employ voluntary choice in selecting their own behaviors. This point of view, called the metaphysical Principle of Determinism, argues that everything that happens, under those particular prevailing conditions, had to happen. Thus, it says that whatever a person did, he or she could not have done otherwise. This means therefore that sinners or Christians are produced by factors over which they have no control, and therefore no responsibility for their behaviors.

Such a psychological view reduces human beings to nothing other than inherited physical bodies that respond to their physical surroundings. Specifically, there is no place in this view for a human spirit that can make independent choices of behaviors. Therefore, this view is not compatible with religion.

There are, as I have said, other psychological views of human nature that are fully harmonious with the Christian thought. For example, the school of Humanistic psychology, championed by psychotherapist Carl Rogers[8], emphasizes a person's ability to make voluntary choices of behaviors on the basis of his or her personal beliefs. This view emphatically does not deny that environmental forces can act upon us to influence our decisions, or that our inherited physical structure is important. It does maintain, however, that we can also at times act according to our chosen beliefs, completely independent of our physical structure and personal training. I suspect that most psychologists, and virtually all non-professionals, subscribe to this Humanistic view.

Because the issue of a viable human will to choose is metaphysical, it is not subject to empirical proof. Therefore, it cannot be proved to exist, *or not to exist*. In the absence of proof one way or another, the acceptance of the concept of a human ability to choose is determined by certain personal characteristics of each person. A person accepts the conviction that makes him or her feel most comfortable.

To be sure, most Christians accept the concept of freedom of choice on the basis of their faith. The Scriptures tell us that God gave us the freedom to make choices. Therefore, for example, we are charged with making selections of holy behaviors over sinful ones.

The main psychological argument in favor of the concept of a viable human will is that it is optimistic.[9] A deterministic view is fatalistic, because it says that we cannot voluntarily make changes to improve our behavior, and therefore we are complete victims of circumstances. In contrast, the belief in freedom of will permits the absolutely vital religious assumption of personal responsibility for one's behaviors. As I have argued previously, our society will be thrown into amoral chaos if our citizens accept the deterministic assumption that they do not have personal voluntary control over their own behaviors.[10] Under a deterministic assumption, each perpetrator of evil would be automatically absolved of blame because he or she could not have chosen to behave in any other way. All people would be placed in the category of people who cannot personally control their own behaviors. For example, we do not consider it possible for very young children, mentally deficient persons or persons with disordered thinking processes to be responsible for their choices of behaviors. Why would we even want to think that everyone was like that? For example, if no one were responsible, teachers could not be blamed for poor teaching, because they would teach only as they had been trained by others. Because no one could be blamed personally for anti-social behaviors, only the behavior itself could be evaluated. No one could be sanctioned, or put in prison; or otherwise punished for misbehavior. Thus, the deterministic view of human psychology cannot solve our social problems.

A major criticism of the assumption of a viable human will is that we do not know how it operates. Indeed, we do not know how it works to influence the operation of our nerves and muscles. This is the familiar mind-body problem. We do not know how a non-material psychological process of mind can influence the material, physical processes of body. Nevertheless, I believe that the viable will is mediated by a non-material spirit of the human being.[11] This spirit influences the human body in some unknown way.

Those who deny the existence of spirits and viable will must try to account for our novel, unpredictable responses in some different way. As I have argued, these proposals involve physical mechanisms which are just as mysterious as the workings of a human spirit.[12] For example, an unpredictable mutation of personal habits is no better understood than is a voluntary choice of behavior.

The answer that science cannot provide can nevertheless be provided by faith. Faith needs no justification for believers. For non-believers the only justification is practical. As I have argued, behavioral scientists can test the psychological and social value, if not the truth, of the belief in viable will.[13] Therefore, if your faith alone is not enough to justify your belief, there is a valid practical argument.

There are many examples of such benefit. For example, such belief is crucial for certain types of psychotherapy.[14] Moreover, it is a critical component in the accordance of human dignity to other persons.[15] That is, one places more value on a person whom you perceive as having the ability to make personal choices, and who makes good choices. Because people are likely to help people that they perceive as having personal dignity, or worth, anything that promotes human dignity fosters helping behaviors. And, that surely is much desired for our society.

Unfortunately, I have heard many Christians rail against the theory of Humanism, as a bad thing. But, the Humanistic view is merely critically deficient from a Christian point of view. It is nevertheless the best psychological theory especially because it is the only psychological theory that is compatible with Christian thinking.

So, we must recognize our human nature. It is human to make choices. The Christian should understand that, and also understand that the basis of his or her choices should be the model established by Jesus Christ. This thinking goes beyond psychology and philosophy, and achieves holiness.

Holey, Wholly, Holy

The above argument indicates that there is no basis for the allegation that the science of psychology does not permit Christian beliefs. Rather, the most effective approach to a science of behavior, in my view, complements and also supplements our religious convictions.

The progression of the appropriate psychological-theological perspective on human beings is given by the following trilogy of terms: Holey, wholly, holy. The first two of these terms refer to the two purely psychological conceptions of human beings: a deficient psychological view and a satisfactory psychologically holistic view. The third—holy—view includes also the spiritual nature of human beings.

The Non-Person

The Behavioristic and Psychoanalytic views in psychology offer a holey conception of human beings, because they deny the capability of people to make free choices of their responses. With gaps in the theory, they cannot account for all of the phenomena of human behaviors, as I have discussed elsewhere.[16]

The Behavioristic and Psychoanalytic views are thus incompatible with the assumption of a spiritual life. Therefore, these theories leave a hole in the conception of human beings.

The Whole Person

The Humanistic approach to psychology is consistent with religious thinking, although it is not itself religious. Humanistic psychology stresses the importance of the individuality, the personhood, the wholeness of every human being. This added characteristic of the whole person is the ability to make choices. An adult human being has the ability at times to choose his or her behaviors independently of heredity and environment.

This conception of people views the character of the person as among the causes of behaviors rather than some external or internal characteristic of the environment, or some manipulation of the environment. This view presumes that a person can make a choice of his or her personal beliefs or convictions, which naturally produce the behaviors associated with those convictions. This is an optimistic view of people because it says that people are not at the complete mercy of circumstances.

The Virtuous Person

The religious approach presumes that the whole person freely chooses virtue. It proposes that the human being is not fully complete—holy—until he or she is endowed, or indwelled, with a spiritual essence. This holy view does not deny the human nature of human beings, but affirms it. It says that Humanism is acceptable to Christian thinking, for example, if it does not represent some end point of thinking about people. It recognizes the true human nature of people, and also affirms that human beings do not necessarily behave like other animals. We human beings indeed have the potential to behave like we are a little lower than the angels, made in the image of God.

Christian training and education, along with a searching of the soul, help us to develop this human potential for holiness. Therefore, a committed Christian is a virtuous person, a holy person, dedicated to a relationship with God that is the source of ethical behaviors. Only a virtuous person can produce ethical behaviors, because such behaviors cannot come from robots, or from people following rules like robots. Virtuous behaviors come from people who choose and strive toward perfection.

The Bible emphasizes the human choice between good and evil. Sometimes the choice is easy, and sometimes not. The words of Paul indicate how difficult the correct choice can be at times:

> We know that the law is spiritual; but I am unspiritual, sold as a slave to sin. I do not understand what I do. For what I want to do I do not do, but what I hate I do. And as I do what I do not want to do, I agree that the law is good. As it is, it is no longer I myself who do it, but it is sin living in me. I know that nothing good lives in me, that is, in my sinful nature. For I have the desire to do what is good, but I cannot carry it out. For what I do is not the good I want to do; no, the evil I do not want to do—this I keep on doing. Now if I do what I do not want to do, it is no longer I who do it, but it is sin living in me that does it.
>
> So I find this law at work: when I want to do good, evil is right there with me. For in my inner being I delight in God's law, but I see another law at work in the members of my body, waging war against the law of my mind and making me a prisoner of the law of sin at work within my members.
>
> What a wretched man I am! Who will rescue me from this body of death? Thanks be to God—through Jesus Christ our Lord!
>
> So then I myself in my mind am slave to God's law, but in the sinful nature a slave to the law of sin.[17]

The important point for us to understand is that we can, and do, make choices. These choices reflect our natures as Christians, or not as Christians. The psychotherapists emphasize that the ability to make good choices, and to be able to associate those choices with the direct consequences, is an indication of good mental health.

Psychology of Ethical Decisions

The discussion of the psychological perspective on Christian living begins with some psychological fundamentals about the production of behaviors. The general formula is: performance = habit x motivation. Thus, to produce Christian behavior (i.e., performance), a person must possess both the habit (capability) for performing Christian behavior, and also the motivation to behave like a Christian. Conventional mathematics tells us that any amount of something multiplied by zero equals nothing. Therefore, when a person has a zero amount of either one of these (i.e., habit or motivation) at any given time, he or she will not perform that behavior.

Practice is required in order to develop the habit sufficiently well so that you can use it effectively when needed. Therefore, to be able to make Christian decisions, you must have practice in choosing Christian responses. For example, suppose that I try to juggle some items to entertain you. I would do a very poor job of juggling, because I have not seriously practiced it. You do not become a juggler without practicing.

The same principle is true for Christian behavior. Such behavior is a skilled response of a different kind. You must train yourself in the habit of Christian responding so that the behavior is available to you when you want it. It does not make sense for you to practice un-Christian responses until you are desperate, and then pray for skill to do the right thing.

You might hear a friend or neighbor say, "I can't make a Christian decision. I never made one before." Of course, he or she is not likely to perform this skilled response any more than he or she can juggle without practice. Admittedly, the Holy Spirit can inspire a person to do Christian things at any time, but for most of us, most of the time, we must work and strive to become more Christ-like. I do not think that God expects us to sit on our hands, and close our minds, passively waiting for His Divine Spirit to take hold of us, to perform Christ-like behaviors in miraculous ways just when we need them.

From all of the possible responses in a given situation, the decision about which one is the Christian one is determined by the will of God for the person in that situation. The Christian nature of the act lies in the ultimate goal, the intended outcome for the behavior. For example, the actual overt act of giving money to a person or organization can be Christian or un-Christian, depending upon the donor's expectations about the good things that the money will buy, in contrast to a hope for selfish personal recognition. Skill, developed through practice, is required to make the discrimination.

If you are skilled enough to perform the Christian act, then you must have sufficient desire to do the right thing. Without the firm desire to be Christian, you will not make the Christian response. For example, consider a task that I can perform very well: tying my shoelace. I have to want to tie my lace at a particular time for it actually to happen. My shoelace will not tie itself. And, I do not consider it appropriate to pray to God to tie it for me.

Therefore, you will not perform the Christian response if you really do not want to be a Christian in that situation at that moment. You may have a stronger motivation to make a different response, say, of revenge or personal glory. It is a crucial choice.

One must be sensitive to the aspects of the total situation—what conditions exist in the environment—that tell us that a Christian response is needed. Discrimination among situations or conditions is therefore required, because different habits are evoked by different environmental contexts. If you do not notice that the needs for Christian responses are present, there is a substantial decrease in the chances for you to manifest the appropriate Christian behaviors.

To be sure, God is always there, always reaching out to us. But, we may not hold up our end of the relationship for one reason or another. For example, we may harden our hearts to His truth at any given time. Or, we may just ignore Him, taking His love and strength for granted. Or, we can pride ourselves on being saved Christians, certified true believers, and just not feel it necessary to work at being Christian. We can show a pride, bordering on arrogance, by assuming that, being Christian, we will automatically do the Christian thing, or—worse—that whatever we do is Christian. This assumption probably represented the thought that was feared by the person who asked to be protected from virtuous people. The person obviously was referring to professed virtue. It is entirely foolish to wish to be protected from truly virtuous people.

Silvis warned us about the sin of assuming that spiritually we are finished products.[18] He pointed out that it was as foolish to say, "I was saved," naming a specific date, as though it were a completed process, as it would be for a child to come home after the first day of kindergarten and announce that he or she had finished his or her education. Silvis said:

> Now, I have said the aim of a growing Christian is to move toward perfection. Maybe you have heard a commencement speaker say, 'You are receiving a diploma, but do not assume you are educated. Learning is a continuing process.' Similarly, the Christian will never stop growing, and will never receive his diploma on this side of eternity.[19]

We must be sensitive to the presence of issues before us that can be resolved in Christian or in non-Christian ways. For example, on several occasions I have been involved in disputes with the Christian leadership within the church about which is the Christian way to handle a given issue. Surely, only a very lucky church member has never been in such a situation. I am not referring to trivial matters, such as placement of the flowers on the altar table, or the type of footwear worn by the pastor. So, for serious ethical dilemmas, how can both parties be correct if they are both committed Christians?

I submit that the person endowed with the Holy Spirit does not fail to notice that there is a problem when someone simply assumes—perhaps even proclaims—that the person with a different opinion obviously has a poorer relationship to God. That callous attitude entails the very sin of pride that was shown by the Pharisee who thanked God that he was not a sinner like the tax collector. Rather, the true believer refers to God's ethical guidelines, as discussed in Chapter 5. And, then, he or she takes a stand. But, remember that the Christian's decisions are empowered, but not necessarily sacred.

Summary

This chapter has argued that a whole person can make voluntary decisions that transcend his or her heredity and environmental experiences. The decisions will be Christian if the person is both virtuous and courageous. This view represents an intersection of psychological and religious thinking. It means that virtuous behaviors will make life better for everyone here on earth.

Notes

1. E. Rae Harcum, *A Psychology of Freedom and Dignity* (Westport, CT: Praeger, 1994).
2. E. Rae Harcum, *Biblical Guidance and Human Choices*, ed. E. Rae Harcum (Williamsburg, VA: Cape Books, 1999).
3. Holy Bible, New International Version (Grand Rapids, MI: Zondervan Publishing House, 1973), Psalm 32: 9-11.
4. Holy Bible, Joshua 24: 14-15.
5. Holy Bible, Galatians 5: 13.
6. Sigmund Freud, *An Outline of Psychoanalysis*, trans. J. Strachey (New York: Norton, 1949).
7. Burrhus F. Skinner, *Science and Human Behavior* (New York: Macmillan, 1953).
8. Carl R. Rogers, A theory of therapy, personality, and interpersonal relationships, as developed in the client-centered framework. In *Psychology: A Study of a Science,* Vol. 3, ed. Sigmund Koch (New York: McGraw-Hill, 1959), 184-256
9. Harcum, *A Psychology of Freedom and Dignity.*
10. *ibid.*
11. *ibid.*
12. E. Rae Harcum, Behavioral paradigm for a psychological resolution of the free will issue, *Journal of Mind and Behavior,* 12, (1991), 93-114. Harcum, *A Psychology of Freedom and Dignity.*
13. E. Rae Harcum, Defensive reactance of psychologists to a metaphysical foundation for integrating different psychologies. *The Journal of Psychology,* 122, (1998), 217-235. E. Rae Harcum, The relative utility of complementary disparate views on voluntarism and determinism. *The Journal of Psychology,* 125, (1990), 217-228. Harcum, Behavioral Paradigm for a psychological resolution.
14. E. Rae Harcum, Barry N. Burijon, and Neill Watson, Client responsibility in the practitioners' operational definition of behavior therapy. *Journal of Human Behavior and Learning,* 5, (1988), 12-16.
15. E. Rae Harcum and Ellen F. Rosen, Perceived dignity as a function of perceived voluntary control of behavior. *Journal of Psychology,* 124, (1990), 495-511. E. Rae Harcum, Ellen F. Rosen, Constance J. Pilkington and Linda C. Petty, An external validation of laboratory evidence for earned dignity. *Journal of Applied Social Psychology, 25*, (1995), 1204-1213.
16. Harcum, *A Psychology of Freedom and Dignity.*
17. Holy Bible, Romans 7: 14-25.
18. Merle Silvis, Ethics in the church. In *Biblical Guidance and Human Choices*, ed. E. Rae Harcum (Williamsburg, VA: Cape Books, 1999), 27-33.

19. *ibid*, 28

Chapter 8

Religion and the Triune Brain

As we try to understand the nature of human beings, we cannot ignore the fact that God has given us bodies, with controlling brains. Further, God has endowed those bodies and brains with certain marvelous physical characteristics. The manner in which we have developed the brains that God has given us determines to a great extent how we behave—how we make our choices of behaviors. But, the fact that we make decisions by involving our brains does not eliminate a non-material, spiritual element as part of the total process. In fact, I assert that such a spiritual component does affect the functioning of the human brain in some unknown way.

Again, this is not to say that the physical brain is not very important to us. In fact, human beings have the largest brains of all land animals with respect to the size of their bodies. Therefore, we actually have more brain to develop and control than other animals. This means that human beings have the highest capacity to make rational decisions, but also we have more difficult decisions to make because we must choose from so many more of the possible responses that are available to humans.

The discussion of the role of brain structure begins with a description of the three major parts of the vertebrate brain.[1] For convenience, I call them the low, middle and high parts. These three parts are like three separate brains, or mentalities, within one body, although they interact intimately and mutually with one another.

The lowest part of the brain, or brain stem, lying just above the spinal cord, is called the vital center, because this part keeps us alive by controlling our eating, drinking, breathing and so forth. Thus, it is vital to the survival of the individual. For example, when we say that a human being is "brain dead," because of some disease or injury, we are referring only to the two higher parts of the brain. Although the low part may require some kind of mechanical support system to maintain the viability of the person, it still must be functioning at some level of effectiveness for the person to be alive. Of course, the so-called brain-dead person is nevertheless still alive.

The middle part of the brain is important in the expression of emotions. Love, hate and rage are made more intense and coordinated by this part of the brain.

The highest part of the brain may be described as a "thinking cap" because it makes most of the learned associations or connections among life events. It is responsible for the most complicated and productive aspects of the tasks of learning, memory and thinking.

Vertebrates that are more primitive than human beings have different relative sizes of the three parts, compared to humans, as well as generally smaller brains. For example, the low part of an alligator brain is the largest part of it and the high part of the alligator brain is the smallest part. This means obviously that alligators are not very good at learning and thinking, but very effective at maintaining the basic (instinctive) behaviors that keep them alive.

This size relationship among the brain parts is completely reversed in humans. That is, humans have a relatively small low brain, but a very large high brain This means that human daily activities necessarily involve a lot more than just competition to stay alive, but it also means that we humans can be much more innovative in our struggle to survive. Humans depend upon the high brain for developing our human capabilities to adapt to our environment. Indeed, we survive because we have a big brain, especially a large high brain, which obviously is more important for our survival in the modern world than having an effective low brain or big teeth and claws. In fact, the functional capacity to love and to care for others is more important for human survival than the weaponry of a big tooth for defending against or for defeating enemies. This is a most important principle to keep in mind for the welfare of our society.

But there is a cost of having the larger high brain. The high part of our brain is not very functional at birth, because it is not developed, and the activity of the small lower brain is not sufficient to keep the newborn human baby alive without outside help. Therefore, the human baby must be cared for by others, usually the parents, while the higher parts of its brain are slowly being developed to take personal control later as the individual matures. So, love and caring by others are important for the survival of human beings, even at the very beginning of life.

There are parallels between the relative sizes of these brain parts and the actual development of individual animals. For example, a lower animal with a simpler brain, like an alligator, is concerned primarily with the vegetative functions of staying alive. The alligator is not capable of much learning because of its small high brain. That means that it is mostly stimulus-bound, such that it tends to respond to environmental stimuli in an unlearned or instinctive manner. To be sure, the effectiveness of this vital activity is natural because the alligator's low brain is relatively large. Thus, the alligator at birth is very good at survival in an alligator world. The neonatal alligator can cope with life on its own about as well as it can as an adult, except for the differences in size and strength. Appropriate routines and rituals of vital responding are built into its very brain structure. Although the alligator is not very good at learning to change its behavior in order to cope with the exigencies of life, it does not need such adaptability to survive, because it is born having the very abilities that it needs the most.

As a consequence, the alligator is very selfish because that is the way it survives. Because of the small high brain, which serves social functions, it is not concerned about social niceties, and getting along with fellow alligators. The alligator says, in effect, "I've got to get mine. I have to eat whatever I can eat whenever I can." Therefore, alligators will even eat their own young. They are deceptive; they are predatory. They survive in an alligator-eat-alligator world.

Unfortunately, there are some people in this world who think and act like they have alligator brains, although their human brains have much greater potential. These people have not properly developed the higher parts of their brains, which contain the God-given potential for adaptability and caring. Whereas the alligators have no choice, these people make bad choices. We will come back later to a discussion of the cause of such alligator mentalities of some humans.

The brain of the cat is structurally between that of the alligator and the human. In the cat, the emotional part of the brain is relatively larger than in the alligator. Still the highest part of the cat brain is not relatively as large as in humans. This means that the cat has emotions that the alligator does not have, and thus it has the capacity to show concern and caring for others. Surely, we have no real concern that the cat will eat its newborn kittens. Rather, she will typically fight ferociously to protect them. The cat can learn and reason better than the alligator, but not as well as the human.

In our house, the cat will stay out of the way of the dog, unless she has new kittens. Then, the dog had better stay away from the kittens. Thus, there are emotional bonds between cat and kittens that are important to the preservation of the species. The newborn kittens, in order to survive, need at first the environmental protection and nurturance of a parent. They cannot even open their eyes for over a week after they are born. But, the adult cat has a sufficient amount of high brain to care for them and to protect them.

The best brain of the vertebrates is human. It is often called the computer brain. To call it a computer brain sounds a bit inhuman, but actually the opposite is true. We must think about the high part of the mature human brain as a large thinking component that is sitting at the top of a complete, complex and integrated brain. This marvelous brain is largely responsible for certain distinctly human characteristics.

The high brain is relatively the largest part which, when fully developed, controls the lower parts of the brain. For example, this so-called thinking cap can control the emotions in social behaviors. It can, in turn, be influenced by the emotions and on occasion actually be overpowered by the emotions. When the computer brain is dominated by the lower parts of the brain, the person behaves like an alligator. This is what Paul was talking about in Romans 7, when he said that often he did what he did not choose to do.

Because the high brain can control the low part, we humans need not be selfish and predatory like the alligator. Need I say that Christianity implies psychological maturity in humans?

Thus, the interactions among these three different parts of our total brain mean that human beings have the capabilities to act like alligators, or to act like cats or, of course, to act like human beings. Because we all have an alligator-like part in our brains, we have to be concerned about controlling the alligator impulses within us. Mature human beings keep the lower parts of the brain under sufficient control for making rational voluntary decisions, whereas the immature brain acts like an alligator brain. The high part of the Christian brain is even more highly developed for serving others.

Now, the difficulty for human parents and mentors is that the very young human brains basically function like alligator brains. The thinking cap of the computer brain does not fully function when the child is born, because it has not been developed by the experience of living in the world. Therefore, the low part of the brain is in control, and the newborn child is as selfish as an alligator. In the maturing child, the highest part of the brain slowly learns to control the survival motivations and social emotions produced by the two lower parts of the brain. In a sense, it takes a little while for the human child to start acting a bit like a human being.

Even in the adult person, there are times when efficient functioning of the lower parts of the brain is necessary and useful, as in some immediate life-threatening crises. For example, a mature human being when threatened with bodily injury by some vicious animal may need to give up control by the thinking cap, and resort to control by the lower parts of its brain in order to survive. But, such impulses can at other times be detrimental to the individual's welfare when the motivations are totally and consistently self-serving, and the emotions are unbridled.

The computer brain sometimes makes up excuses for those times when it is not in control. We psychologists have technical names for such occurrences; they are called defense mechanisms, which keep the person from recognizing the anti-social nature of certain behaviors. For example, the thinking brain can rationalize stealing another person's bread because, it argues, the bread would only make the other person fat.

The feeling that one is in control of one's life is a major component of mental health. This feeling is developed by experiencing successes in controlling one's selfish urges through efficient functioning of the thinking cap. Each mature and Christian response builds confidence in the person's ability to control un-Christian motivations. For example, as we serve others, we prove to ourselves that we are not like alligators, dominated by our emotions and our selfish impulses. The selfish impulses that are so important for survival to the alligator, are likely to interfere with the social adjustment of the human being, and thus ironically damage chances for success and survival.

Moreover, the control of impulsive behavior will tend to prevent a person from putting himself or herself in uncomfortable and stressful situations. Such control will also help the person deal with stressful crises. Success in control breeds further successes.

Brain, Moral Behavior and Virtue

The physiology of the three levels of the brain parallels very nicely the developmental theory of moral behavior proposed by Lawrence Kohlberg.[2] He proposed six stages in moral development, broken down into three levels. The first level, called pre-conventional morality, represents the first two stages, in which the child is dominated by selfish interests and practical issues in relating to others. At this level, the child is motivated toward, first, avoiding punishment, and, second, gaining reward. This type of morality can be recognized as alligator-brained, because the 'right' response is merely the one that is rewarded (i.e., successful), and the 'wrong' response is the one that is punished (i.e., not successful). It is indeed selfish, and thus not Christian.

The second moral level of Kohlberg, conventional morality, also entails two stages. The child in the first stage of this level seeks to gain the approval of others and to avoid their disapproval. In the second stage, the child adopts the code of the group about rules and order, in order to fulfill his duty to the group. Thus, the child understands what is conventional and expected by the group, but still not the concept of right and wrong, in the sense of good and not good. The child is therefore moral, socialized by the particular society, because he or she conforms to social norms. But, he or she is not yet ethical. Thus, the morality is legalistic, as evidenced by the saying "I'm a law-abiding citizen." This is still not yet Christian behavior.

Kohlberg's third level of moral development, the level of post-conventional morality, is based on principles of right and justice. In the first stage at this level, the individual's decisions are based on the rights, values and principles that are perceived to promote the public welfare. In the second stage, the person is guided, in Kohlberg's words, by abstract "universal ethical principles" which have become part of his or her own personal code of conduct. Therefore, the thinking of an individual on the third level transcends rules and laws as governors of his or her behavior. He or she believes that just laws should be obeyed, and unjust laws disobeyed. Thus, a person who achieves this post-conventional morality responds to higher principles of behavior than adherence to group norms of behavior.

The thinking cap must identify and develop these ideas of ethical behavior. A person who has achieved this level of morality understands the ethical concepts of right and wrong, which transcend mere group norms of thinking. The final stage of true ethical reasoning, said Kohlberg, has been achieved by only a few persons, such as Mahatma Ghandi and Dr. Martin Luther King, Jr.

In his later writing, Kohlberg raised doubts that there is actually such a distinctive sixth state. He suggested that moral development stops at some advanced version of the fifth stage, which is based on concepts of justice for the public good.

What about Christian behaviors? Kohlberg recognized one more stage of development beyond his six stages of moral development, which he called a "Stage Seven." This is not just another moral stage, but a truly ethical stage. A person at this stage is fundamentally grounded in issues of justice, but integrates those principles into personal answers to questions about the meaning of life and death. Thus, the person rises above simple moral questions that may be resolved by purely rational methods. The highest ethical development cannot be reached by logic and reason alone, but by "contemplative experience." Such experience can be described in theological terms as a "union with God," or "atonement"—

the process of becoming one with God. It is, of course, Christian.

According to Kohlberg, identification or union with a deity begins with the despair that arises as we realize our own mortality and insignificance as self-oriented creatures. We resolve this despair, not by science or logic, but by changing our perspective from human and worldly principles to a higher order and more harmonious perspective on life. This sense of unity, with a higher perspective on life, must be *achieved* by personal experience and contemplation. A person in Stage Seven perceives a loving God to be the ultimate reality of life, and thus he or she becomes holy in outlook. I note that this holy outlook cannot be given by another; it requires personal striving and achievement.

This search for atonement is also initiated by God, who reaches for us, just as we reach for Him. Atonement is therefore a mutual achievement. This higher perspective on life is expressed by the Greek word "agape'," which means responsible, selfless, sacrificial, unconditional "love" or "charity," extended to all, including one's enemies as an act of grace, without regard for merit. Therefore, the spiritual union with God implies selfless love and service to other human beings, according to a standard that goes beyond duty and justice. The fruits of agape' are acts of grace, from God to humans, and from one human to another. Therefore, the human animal has the capacity to overcome, or transcend, the selfish tendencies that are characteristic of the lowest animals, and to act according to the image of God, revealed in Jesus Christ, the perfect Model.

Role of Learning

The above discussion emphasizes the need to give instruction to children to help them move from one stage of moral behavior to a higher one. In his early writings, Kohlberg concluded that moral values could not be shaped by indoctrination and advocacy, but only by actual discussion of moral issues. Later, he recanted that view, and firmly stated that parents and educators should teach the proper conduct and behaviors to children in order to help the youngsters advance to the higher levels of morality and ethics.

I agree with the expert. Our Christian ethics affirm and incorporate the highest moral principles, and they also add to these principles the fullness of responsible love as revealed in the New Testament. The highest ethics incorporates Christian standards. The questions go beyond the stages of "What is everybody else doing?" to "What should I be doing with God's help, according to a Christian model, in order to become perfect, as the Scriptures instruct?"

The issue for us all is whether anybody really achieves the ability to respond to such higher principles, or whether they only follow rules for behavior. This is an important point because the difference distinguishes the Old Testament and the New Testament. The Old Testament provided rules for us. But Jesus used a new approach. The rich, young ruler said, in essence, "I followed all the rules, now what more do I need." Jesus said, basically, "There is something more that you need, because you missed the whole point of the new, great law." Therefore, we cannot follow a list of rules, and thus satisfy our ethical problems. There must be understanding with love. Works—good deeds—alone will not satisfy. The people of God must respond by understanding the Word, knowing Christ, and not by blindly following halter lines like the domestic animals, in the form of rules laid down by secular leaders, guided by science alone.

Jesus presented a new approach. He said that we need to be concerned about the spirit of God rather than any specific rules. So, He gave us the Great Commandment. This is not just a rule, but also a guideline for living, a guiding principle that requires some interpretation when translated into daily modern life.

Matthew gives an amplification of the charge to love our neighbor, as follows:

> Ye have heard that it hath been said thou shalt love thy neighbor and hate thine enemy, but I say unto you, love your enemies, bless them that curse you, do good to them that hate you and pray for them which despitefully use you and persecute you, that ye may be the children of your Father which is in heaven, for He maketh His sun to rise upon the evil and on the good and sendeth rain on the just and on the unjust. . . . Be ye therefore perfect, even as your Father which is in heaven is perfect.[3]

The charge to be perfect is not just a rule. It is a guideline and requires a proper spirit for interpretation and for action. How do we know what it is to be perfect in terms of real life situations? We must learn what it takes to be perfect in the eyes of God. We have to use our thinking cap, the highest part of our human brain, to develop a concept of perfection that is usable for us. We learn what is right (correct) behavior first from rewards in the environment in the earlier stages of our moral development and, of course, from imitation of others—particularly our parents. This is why human models are so important. Children are learning from models all of the time. Parents must hold up Christ as the ultimate model. One alternative to understanding model behavior is the life of an alligator.

There is always another, different model out there, of course. That model may promote behaviors that are un-Christian, like the alligator. Therefore, you must teach your children what you want them to know. And you must model Christian behaviors in your life, and reward the children only for making the desired Christian responses. That will give them an ethical, virtuous thinking cap, like a mature, developed human adult.

Ethical Categories

The same learning principles that cover the acquisition of Christian behaviors also apply to immoral behaviors and for unethical behaviors. In this experiential way the child learns what is, and is not, admired by the parents. And so the child categorizes the world; experience tells the child what is good, what is bad, etc. The same is also true for older children and adults. What the models whom we admire tell us about proper behaviors is very important to us. This is the way that we develop our high brains.

Many years ago I did research with some rats in which, soon after birth, I restricted their experience of locomotion in different planes.[4] For example, I had some rats that only traveled horizontally and could not climb up and down. Later, I found that the rats who had been living in the horizontal environment had problems learning to choose between up versus down paths to find food. I argued that they were deficient in the development of the concepts of up and down and, therefore, these concepts were not as readily available for use when they were needed in, say, learning to find food.

Similarly, other psychological research has shown that enhanced sensory stimulation improves the cognitive performance of human infants. Therefore, if a child does not have the appropriate ethical experiences to install the concepts of right and wrong into his or her thinking cap, so that he or she can know what behaviors represent the right and wrong, then the child cannot use these concepts later when he or she needs them to make ethical decisions. So, if the capacity to make ethical decisions has not been developed, we do not have the power to choose wisely, simply because we have not developed that power. And then we may act like alligators, stuck in total control by our low brain.

To achieve the highest level of ethical reasoning means that we have to transcend the conventional—what other people are doing—and use our own developed categories of right and wrong in organizing our understanding of the world. Our categories should be based on our personal understanding of the will of God.

We must be extremely careful whenever we use other people's categorizations of life events. For example, let us consider the very controversial issue of abortion. The pro-choice people say that a woman's body is her own. Well, that is surely true. Using that labeling category, you respond that a woman should have control of her own body; therefore, you say "Yes" to abortion. On the other side, the pro-life people say, "Abortion is murder." This is another labeling category. Using that category, you say, "Wait a minute, I don't believe in murder;" therefore, you say "No" to abortion. Whose category should you use? The only reasonable answer to this question is: establish your own categories in thinking, based on your own understanding from your Christian heritage. Do not use someone else's categories.

We all must make our own discriminations and establish our own categories, based on the criterion of love, and not let some less knowledgeable or less loving neighbors tell us how to make ethical decisions based on how *they* categorize or organize the world. The ultimate model is Jesus Christ, not some group norm established by a group of citizens on earth.

I find it difficult to organize the world neatly. For example, it seems to me that the ethics of abortion depend a great deal upon the circumstances. Surely, abortion as a method of birth control is ethically wrong. On the other hand, the future—perhaps even the life—of a young mother may be saved by an abortion. A fertilized egg undoubtedly has life. But, in my view, it does not have personhood. I do not presume to suggest by what age a fetus has developed its own personhood. Nevertheless, I think that the distinction between a fetus and a person is important. And surely, the mother is mature enough to be a person.

I have a couple of examples of the ethical inconsistencies that one encounters in life. Briefly during the Vietnam War, I was a visiting scholar at the University of California, Berkeley. The free speech movement had started at Berkeley. But, how do you define free speech? I heard the story of how a man opposed to what they were doing at one free speech rally was refused access to the microphone. This is an example of a logic-tight compartment. Does the right of free speech depend upon who owns the microphone? How would a Christian decide?

Rigid rules really do not help us here. When I was chairman of the Virginia Board of Psychologists' Examiners, the state board for the licensing of professional psychologists, in order to satisfy the lawyers, we had to write rules to describe the bases for our decisions. These rules were derived to determine which candidates for licensing as psychologists would be approved to offer psychological services to the public. These rules had the power of law. Now, the problem about rules is how to interpret them. For example, one rule was that a person was required to have a certain number of college graduate courses containing specified content in psychology. Some candidates showed up with their lawyers, asking, "What is an academic course? Does writing a doctoral thesis give you credit for a college course? Is a directed-reading tutorial the same as a course?" What is your definition? Here is the example I think is best of all: we told one man that to be licensed he must take a course in Physiological Psychology. He took the course, but he never took the final examination. He came back with his lawyers and said, "You said to take a course in physiological psychology; you didn't say I had to pass it!" Our lawyers became very nervous over his case, because that is the sort of thing that makes lawyers nervous. Nevertheless, we would not back down on the implicit requirement that taking the course means that it should be satisfactorily completed, meaning the achievement of a passing grade. This implies a reasonable knowledge of the course content, which we thought was necessary. Such examples illustrate the unhappy role of rules and legalism in questions of ethics.

Service on such a licensing board provides a precise example of the type of dilemmas that Christians face every day. The examiner cannot simply express his or her love for the applicants by passing every one. Discriminations must be made. There is, on the one hand, the responsibility of the examiners to protect the people of the state, who have a right to presume that any person who has been licensed is indeed qualified to render the services stipulated on his or her license. That is a form of concern, if not love, for the people.

On the other hand, the examiners have the responsibility to allow a person to earn a livelihood by engaging in the profession for which he or she presumably has prepared by study and appropriate experience. Rules and guidelines having the force of law must be written and approved in order to inform the public about the requirements for licensure in that particular state, and to ensure that the same standards are applied fairly to everyone.

A given issue is often not black or white, clearly ethical or unethical, but represents some shade of gray, requiring a subjective decision to assign it to one category or the other. Thus, there is small wonder that a person makes mistakes.

This sensible and practical approach is the way that the Bible must also be interpreted. Any rule, or implied rule, must be interpreted with sense, as John Wesley understood. Such flexibility is, however, not always the way of the lawyers or the religious fundamentalists, who insist on strict literal interpretations of the Scriptures and formal rules. But, I submit, Christians should view their religious commandments with broad judgment.

Jesus gave the answer to difficult questions in terms of having the right spirit. He never gave a direct answer to a question of the proper behavior under a specific circumstance. He answered with another question, or with parables that required the listener to forge the answer using his or her own background and wisdom. That is the best way to teach. It assumes that the listener has a developed high part in his or her brain.

The Christian questioner will not craft the correct answer, if he or she is not seeking God's truth. This assertion is supported by a verse from Psalms: "The fear of the Lord is the beginning of wisdom, all who follow his precepts have good understanding. To him belongs eternal praise."[5]

Therefore, we must open ourselves to receive the right spirit—the spirit of God. There is assurance that it is available to us, but not that we will accept it, you see. We have to strive for it. If we have the right spirit, then our decisions will transcend mere rules and ascend to the highest planes and reaches of ethical development. If we do not have the right spirit, then valid answers are not likely. Obviously, we must first decide which path we wish to take, as discussed in Chapter 3. Jesus made it very clear that a person cannot serve two masters.

Conclusion

The task for the behavioral technologist, to program the person to make just the correct response to the particular stimulus configuration, is obviously impossible, except in the most simple of life situations. Clearly, the best way to ensure that a given person will make the pro-social response in a given situation is to ensure as best one can that he or she is a virtuous person. Only the virtuous, or holy, person will have developed concepts such as agape', of a selfless love, that can be applied appropriately in all circumstances under all conditions. Such a virtuous person is produced by religious training and education.

R. S. Peters quoted a psychoanalyst as saying that, psychologically speaking, what we call reason means saying, "No," to oneself.[6] This means that sometimes the reasonable, sensible thing for us to do is to follow the guidance of our better judgment, coming from the computer part of our brain. Then, we will resist responding to the impulses from the lower parts of our brain, those that impel us toward the self-gratification and self-love of the alligator. Therefore, we must strive to follow the dictates of the highest part of our brains which are telling us when a pleasure is sinful or dangerous, telling us to say, "No," to the commands of the lower parts of the brain which seek pleasures of the flesh.

I want to add that I think Christianity is the best policy—that ethics is the best policy from a practical sense, as well as from a religious one. Even though it may appear that alligator behavior will foster survival through personal gain, in the long run alligator behavior for humans is self-defeating. I personally think that "what goes around comes around." I do not think that there is a perfectly just world, but I do think that God has ordained the principles that control our universe. He does not always need to punish the evil-doer, because the evil that one does typically brings its own appropriate punishment. For example, a person who spends time watching pornography is not spending time doing something useful to benefit himself or herself, by developing his or her thinking cap. This principle reflects one of God's natural laws.

Therefore, I think that God's plan for us is best. When the highest part of the brain is saying, "No", to the lower parts, it is saying, "Yes", to itself. Instead of being enslaved to the goals of the lower brain, the thinking cap is then free to realize its own potential for personal growth, intellectual and social satisfactions and useful service to society. The person is empowered to behave like a Christian, sharing love, and giving it and receiving it. Instead of behaving like the lowest animals, a person can fulfill God's wish for him or her to be just a little lower than the angels. And that surely represents the best of mental health, as God intended.

Notes

1. P. D. Maclean, The imitative-creative interplay of our three mentalities. In *Astride Two Cultures*, ed. H. Harris (London: Hutchinson, 1979), 187-213.
2. Lawrence Kohlberg, Revisions in the theory and practice of moral development. In *New Directions for Child Development*, ed. W. Damon (San Francisco: Jossy-Boss, 1978). Lawrence Kohlberg, *Essays on moral development: Vol 1. The Philosophy of Moral Development* (San Francisco: Harper & Rowe, 1981).
3. Holy Bible, New International Version (Grand Rapids, MI: Zondervan Publishing House, 1973), Matthew 5: 43-45, 48.
4. E. Rae Harcum, Exploring and learning in a three-dimensional maze of rats with restricted experience in one dimension. PhD. dissertation, *University of Michigan Microfilms*, Publ. No. 12581, 1955.
5. Holy Bible, Psalm 111: 10.
6. R. S. Peters, *Psychology and Ethical Development* (London: Geo. Allen and Union Ltd, 1974).

PART IV. CHRISTIAN'S COMMITMENT

Chapter 9

The Wages of Virtue

In this chapter, I am referring to the intrinsic wages of virtue, of love itself, and not to any possible wages that are contingent upon good deeds in life. We know that our virtuous beliefs get us into Heaven, and not the praiseworthy deeds that directly result from those beliefs. But, to be sure, a virtuous person will naturally perform good works in his or her life on earth.

The life that is promised to us as a reward for virtue has two forms. The first is a physical form that is to be enjoyed for a limited time on earth. We believe that this physical life will be followed by a spiritual form of life that is to be enjoyed eternally in Heaven. Jesus gave us the promise: "For God so loved the world that he gave his one and only Son, that whoever believes in him shall not perish but have eternal life."[1] Although the exact nature of this Heavenly form of life is a mystery to us, we know that it is greatly to be desired.

The eternal life in Heaven to be expected as the wages of virtue has often been called "The Pie in the Sky." That description indicates some kind of delayed reward for those who are not rewarded on earth for their virtue. I want to get away from such thinking for a moment, and emphasize the earthly rewards of virtue. This does not mean that I am trying to detract in any way from the ultimate goal of the Christian to achieve virtue as the only way to Heaven. I merely assert that a commitment to virtue will also in all likelihood produce prosperity and joy on earth, which is to say mental health.

Christian holiness is not equivalent to simply wearing a hair shirt to produce suffering. When we speak of a Christian as being a suffering servant, we do not mean to imply that a Christian life is one of deliberate unrelieved suffering. In fact, the meaning is quite the contrary. We mean that a Christian is willing to make sacrifices, if necessary, in the service of others. But, the Christian gains joy from the service, because that is what it means to be a Christian.

Moreover, all Christians should strive to secure the same prosperity and joy for everyone on earth, and that includes themselves as a natural fall-out from helping others. In turn, our helping behaviors become witness to the Word to all people to induce them to help also. Therefore, there is an incidental multiple benefit from our helping behaviors.

Eternal Life

In the Beatitudes, Jesus promised us the fruits of Heaven if we obey His commands and endure tribulation for His sake.[2] The descriptions of the rewards for the faithful are very appealing. Indeed, we can experience what Heaven is like only through such descriptions and metaphors in the Bible. In 1 Corinthians, Paul describes Heaven as being perfect and permanent when we put on our spiritual body.[3]

Surely, the actual splendor and joy of Heaven are greater than we can even imagine. The Bible tells us that Heaven is different from anything that we have experienced, wonderful far beyond our earth-bound experience. We can imagine eternal life, although not what it would be like in a different—spiritual—state that we know on earth. We are assured that Heaven is much to be desired, like a pearl of great price, indeed worthy of any price that we might pay.

Earthly Life

There are those who say that confusion and self-deception for Christians are not possible because the Holy Spirit is within us. I disagree, but not because I think that God cannot accomplish all things. I do think that such general preemption of our human choice is not a part of God's plan. I do not think that He would give us the power to choose, and then take it completely away from us when it really counts.

There is evidence all around us that God allows His people to make choices. I contend that it is possible even for a committed Christian to make bad choices—that is, to have momentary lapses into sin. For example, people are not miraculously changed into perfection by joining a church. Joining a church is a giant step toward perfection, to be sure, because a presumed choice for holiness has been made. But, church membership does not forever provide a valid, nonrevocable ticket to Heaven. The ticket must be kept up-to-date, validated almost daily, or otherwise it becomes worthless. Jesus did not instruct us to feed His sheep until we are saved. He said that if you are saved, you will feed His sheep.

Whatever God permits is part of His plan. This assertion is surely not to condone sin, but to acknowledge its existence, even in the church. To deny this truth is to commit the Pharisee Fallacy, which says that church members are too holy to commit sin.

I once heard a rather humorous parable from the pulpit that illustrates the role of human choices and works in God's plan. The story tells how a farmer was describing to his pastor how he had worked to revive and restore an abandoned farm. The farmer bragged, "By a vision of what this place could be, and by tireless hard work, my family and I have turned it into a showplace." The pastor gently corrected him: "You and God have accomplished this miracle." The farmer agreed, "Yes, you are right, Pastor. But, you should have seen what it looked like when God had it by Himself."

So, God's plan is to use us as His instruments and models. We are His hands and His feet on earth. We are the living stones that are needed to build His Kingdom.

Once we have decided what is God's will for us, we must then act resolutely on our decision. We must make ourselves do in our lives what we know we ought to be doing. Often, we devise many rationalizations to justify doing other things. That is truly a real part of being only human, and another pitfall for the person who would be Christian.

It is human nature to experience internal conflicts between our needs for simple selfish pleasures and the pleasures of Christian living. In a sense, it is a war of control between different parts (levels) of our brains, as discussed in the previous chapter. But, we humans also have psychological tools to combat the psychological processes that keep us from following God's road map. These psychological tools, provided for us by the Holy Spirit, include the ability to love, to be sensitive to the needs of others, to make discriminations among similar paths, to learn, to evaluate, to compromise, to relax and to strive to be better. I submit that these are the actual mechanisms by which God executes His promise of personal peace for those who follow Him.

Personal Health and Joy

Psychological thinking would predict that any person who lives a Christian life will reap huge benefits in terms of a happy and productive life within his or her social setting. This is precisely what Christianity offers. Christ does not offer fame and fortune. But, He surely does not promise that Christians will *not* have fame and fortune. Through the Bible, He speaks in terms of states of mind that transcend the physical circumstances of life. A person can be happy and productive without material advantages, just as a person can be miserable despite having more worldly goods and prestige than most of us can imagine. For proof of this statement, I merely refer to current and recent newspapers and television newscasts. Christians understand from the Paradox of Christian Living why some celebrities with seemingly every material advantage in life nevertheless commit suicide in despair, or land in prison or rehabilitation.

The true question concerns what it takes to make the person happy and productive. Most readers of this book, at least, are looking for happiness through something other than wealth and physical possessions. After all, this book is about psychology and Christian living. The readers have not been told that the book will make them successful in the sense that the secular world uses the term. In fact, the book is not appropriate for those who would find happiness only in material ways, except to urge them to change priorities.

When the Christian follows an aphorism such as "Honesty is the best policy," he or she is motivated primarily to do what is right in the eyes of God. The idea is not merely to avoid punishment by the earthly forces of law enforcement. Thus, the Christian who desires health and joy in his or her earthly life is faced with the same paradox as with eternal life.

The practical advantages of a commitment to Christian living can be summarized in several major categories of experiences in life. As examples, we can cite: dealing with bereavement; believing in personal control of one's life; establishing good interpersonal relations; and maintaining a high level of personal mental health. This list of categories is neither exclusive nor exhaustive.

Bereavement

The Christian belief in eternal life is a great psychological comfort during times of bereavement. If there were no other value from a belief in God and heaven, this one must be judged as adequate. The fact that it works is undeniable. I myself have relied on this belief to see me through bereavements many times. I have seen it work for others countless times as well.

But, be sure that the nature of things is that the belief cannot just be hauled out of retirement for spot duty. I do not think that the adoption of a temporary stance of belief during bereavement, while suspending belief at other times, can be effective. The Paradox of Christian Living says that the commitment cannot be embraced simply for personal gain. Belief cannot be turned easily on and off like a water faucet only when you are thirsty.

Frankly, I do not understand how the un-churched and non-religious people manage to endure the loss of a loved one. Christians are comforted because the Bible assures us that Jesus has gone before to prepare a place for our loved ones. I tried to describe my feelings about this promise in a short poem that I wrote a few years ago:

THE GREATEST GIFT

The greatest gift you sent us, Lord,
The morn of Easter did afford,
To comfort us in doleful day,
For mourning o'er the temple clay,
Where lately lived a one adored,
The earthly frame of one adored.

For Thou did prove to all bereft,
That living soul from body cleft,
Though symbol stays, freed spirit soars,
From flesh infirm and chafing chores,
And only crumbling crust is left,
'Tis merely mortal dust is left.

Thy Son in rising did fulfill,
The blissful promise of Thy will,
That joy engulf our instant grief,
For Easter dawn demands belief:
Who followed Jesus, follows still,
On earth who followed, follow still.

Personal Control

A psychological description of the processes in making Christian decisions acknowledges the self-serving, hedonistic urges that originate in the lowest parts of the human brain. These urges must be brought under control by higher centers of the brain. This process of developing control over selfish pleasures parallels the development of both moral behaviors that reflect the ideals of our human society and also Christian behaviors that reflect the will of God.

The virtuous person has gained control over selfish urges. That is the best use of our potential power. Therefore, the best way to induce pro-social behaviors in a person is to develop virtue in that person. Virtue is developed through religious teachings and worship experiences.

No one can program all of the specific appropriate behaviors through psychological technology. One cannot anticipate each of the instances of a virtual infinity of possible life situations. The best insurance, then, is to become a virtuous person, which means to be guided and controlled by the Holy Spirit.

Interpersonal Relations

Christianity can play a major beneficial role in our interpersonal relations. The goal is not just to avoid conflicts. Some conflicts are actually based on love, because the Christian confronts those who perpetrate evil on God's children. Whether or not the Christian is successful in this, he or she nevertheless also helps to bring the kingdom of God upon the earth, because the acts of kindness are actually witnesses of Christian love.

There is a personal gain as well. Psychological research shows that a person who is perceived by others to be voluntarily helping other people tends to be admired by others.[4] The increase in admiration comes because the helper is thus perceived as virtuous. With the increase in admiration comes a host of other favorable human responses to the admired person, such as help and support. The admiration is appropriately lessened, of course, if the admired behavior is perceived as actually motivated by the desire to be admired.

Another personal gain occurs because the expressions of love and caring for others produce happy climates that are associated through learning to the individual responsible for those good feelings. Therefore, the Christian gains in popularity with other people, because people will seek to be a part of his or her happy climate. The Christian does not seek to gain friends through love for them. Yet, personal popularity nevertheless is the result of spreading Christian love. That is the best and surest way to win friends and to influence people.

Love for our lovable neighbors is not difficult. Neither is it difficult to have love and reconciliation for those who have offended us and then asked for forgiveness. But, to love and forgive those who have offended us and not asked for forgiveness is terribly difficult. Nevertheless, we must be reconciled to our neighbors before we can be fully reconciled to God. Such reconciliation to God can be achieved by human beings, if they truly desire it. God offers it as an act of grace to those who will accept it.

Successful marriage, and also the production of successful friendships, can be guided by a Christian approach to life. The approach involves the translation of Christian principles into behaviors designed to preserve the marriage or friendship. All such behaviors can be defended on rational argument, as well as on Christian grounds. Just as Christian love will bring peace on earth among neighbors and friends, it will specifically bring peace in the home.

Mental Health

We cannot make a simple statement that guilt is useful, or that guilt is harmful, to mental health. This is another behavioral paradox, because the influence of guilt on mental health depends on the nature and strength of the guilt. Productive guilt is needed when we have not behaved like Christians. It makes us try to do better.

But, we must not have so much guilt that we become immobilized by it. Guilt can render us incapable of doing the good that we could accomplish if we did not feel so guilty. God asks only for productive guilt. He is willing to forgive our imperfections if we simply strive for perfection.

God does not assure us that we will not die, or that we will not experience some failures and periods of despair in our lives. He does assure us of peace and joy in our lives if we truly love Him and act accordingly toward others. In Galatians, Paul says, "But the fruit of the Spirit is love, joy, peace, long-suffering, gentleness, goodness, faith, meekness, temperance: against such there is no law."[5] Such peace and joy can be experienced in our hearts despite setbacks and stressful hassles coming from our environment. And, peace and joy are also likely to be experienced through positive responses of other people in our environment to our emanations of Christian spirituality and joy.

It is reasonable and reassuring that the empirical research in our modern society does corroborate the truths in the Bible. If it did not, we would have to assume that we were not interpreting the Bible correctly in order to understand its truths. In any case, with respect to mental health, we have surely understood the Bible correctly.

Psychologists have found that those persons who practice religion as a means of achieving certain worldly goals in life are more likely to manifest *fewer* indications of mental health than those who do not practice any religion. I have given these selfish people the names of tinsel lovers and Churchians. They drape themselves in the pretty practices of religion as a means of securing certain secular rewards. For example, they go to church for the social relationships, and to help establish a prestigious place in the community. They appear to pray in order to assume a happy and peaceful life. In a word, it is a selfish practice of religion. And, as we know, Jesus said that such an approach would not be successful in achieving salvation.

The situation is completely happy for what I call committed Christians. These people practice Christianity as an end in itself—the practice of what I have called good religion.[6] Ventis found that good religion is related to good mental health.[7] Good mental health includes such positive factors in life as freedom from worry and guilt, feelings of personal control and competence, feelings of self worth, habits of principled behavior and open-mindedness in personal attitudes.

Those who practice good religion include, of course, committed Christians. Their sole aim is to be virtuous, to follow the Great Commandment, to be perfect as God has commanded. They spend time in private religious thought and meditation. They feel that their prayers in private carry at least as much meaning and emotion as those they say in public religious services. They try to carry their religion over into all of their dealings in life, and use those beliefs to guide them in their whole approach to living. In sum, God is ever with them. Or, they are ever with God.

One reason that committed Christians can enjoy better mental health is because they can forgive. In discussing the need and nature of forgiveness with many people over many months, I have been constantly reminded that the withholding of forgiveness can cost a person dearly in terms of his or her own mental health. Harboring resentment for real or imagined offenses can tragically erode the personal peace and joy. If forgiveness is withheld because there is a lack of love and caring for the other person, then the natural wages are anguish for the possessor of the resentment. It is not necessary to forgive the transgressor overtly, in order to restore personal peace. One must merely give him or her our love and understanding. That seems to me to be the hallmark of a Christian.

Self-actualization

Christian living can count dividends beyond simple mental health. It can help the person to achieve the full potentials that God has endowed. The Humanist psychologist, Abraham Maslow called this a psychological state of "self-actualization," meaning such characteristics as feeling comfortable with one's self and concentrating attention on general social problems, rather than personal problems.[8] Thus, the person who fulfills the ideals of this psychological concept would also fulfill many of the Christian ideals of perfection. A victorious life is a self-actualized one.

Peace

Christians want peace. But, we must know that Christian peace is an inner peace, a peace of the soul. It can occur in the middle of external strife, and even turmoil. Peace comes from the realization that one fights the good fight, runs the good race. We cannot have peace if we pull back from righteous strife.

We also cannot have inner peace if we withhold love for others, particularly if the withholding of love leads to hostile acts against them. Conflicts that are not in the service of the God of Love are simply acts of aggression. They will therefore not lead to peace, either inner or outward.

The bottom line is that healing peace is a gift of God. It cannot be achieved by one human being working alone. There is, I am sure, no corner of the earth, no inner peace of the mind that is so remote from the realities of life that achieving it in a solitary retreat will guarantee peace. Nevertheless, peace is available as a gift from the Lord for those who will merely accept it. Jesus said, "Peace I leave with you, my peace I give unto you: not as the world giveth, give I unto you. Let not your heart be troubled, neither let it be afraid."[9]

Therefore, peace comes from believing in Christ and following Him in our personal life. And, remember, Christian living does not mean avoidance of strife. Inner peace comes from doing God's will, wherever it leads, cost what it may. External peace may be shattered as we attempt to do God's work in the world. We must fight the forces that lead to poverty and hunger, to pollution, to the drafting of unjust laws, to the moral seduction and degradation of our young people. We cannot have inner peace if we see evil in the world and back off.

But, always remember that our motivation must be Christ-based. For behavior thus motivated the inner rewards are great. We begin to show our inner peace as we endeavor to do the will of God, to do His work in the world. His work is to oppose actively those who work against Him, and to spread His love actively to all of His children. Paul made it clear that a peace that passes all understanding is the reward of those who labor for the Lord:

> Finally, brothers, whatever is true, whatever is noble, whatever is right, whatever is pure, whatever is lovely, whatever is admirable—if anything is excellent or praiseworthy—think about such things. Whatever you have learned from me, or seen in me—put it into practice. And the God of peace will be with you.[10]

Thus, we are instructed to work actively on Godly things. We are not instructed simply to refrain from ungodly acts. We must be actively virtuous.

The Christian should not expect that even the combined power of psychological science and religious faith can achieve complete, uninterrupted psychological peace and continuous sublime happiness. Although the word, peace, means to be free from fears, because of conflicts and other aggravations that prevent personal tranquility and interpersonal harmony, we cannot achieve such a desired uninterrupted state on earth. The Scriptures promise us more and longer intervals of peace and joy, rather than continuously uninterrupted peace and joy. Peace and joy for the Christian on earth may last only until the next spiritual decision. Accordingly, the legitimate and appropriate goal of this book is to help the Christian reader achieve peace of conscience and the joy of victory over sin.

So, the promise to us is not that we will have a life free of conflict and strife. The promise is that we will have God's inner peace because of our belief in Him and commitment to His work. We understand that God carries us through the difficult times. That is the peace that passes all human understanding.

In their book, which describes their reactions to their visits to various religious services through the country, Jim Henderson and Matt Casper—a pastor and an atheist, respectively—posed questions to themselves after each service.[11]

One question, after attendance at a service by Joel Osteen in Houston, asks whether or not the main issue for Christians is their belief in an afterlife. The pastor, Jim, answered:

> Not for Casper and not for me. My life with Christ is now. I want to make this world a better place. I want to see Jesus' prayer answered that his Kingdom would come on Earth as it is in heaven. I want to see the kingdoms of this world become the kingdoms of our God and his Christ. I want the incarnate Jesus to express himself through me to the poor in spirit. I want to give a cup of cold water to a little child in Jesus' name and see the five loaves and two fish of my life multiplied to feed people who are looking to discover a God who truly likes them. Going to heaven is icing on the cake, and I expect Jesus' first words to me upon arrival to simply be 'Nice try.'[12]

Surely, a Christian who confidently expects for God to say in the end, "Nice try," would enjoy the most sublime peace on Earth.

Benefits to Society

Society directly benefits when Christians emphasize both of the two faces of the Great Commandment. The first face deals with a Christian's relation to God. The other face deals with a Christian's relationship to society. Obviously, the second is dependent on the first. In fact, there are those who say that the second half of the Great Commandment is redundant with the first, and is therefore unnecessary. But, obviously Jesus thought it was necessary to include it.

Jesus' reason for including the second part of the Great Commandment provides the main theme for this book: To emphasize that a person who loves God must show such love through works which reflect that love. In a word, Jesus said that if you love Him, you must feed His lambs. James reiterated the message: there is no faith without the works that spring from that faith. An emphasis on the second face is necessary for practical reasons, because the world is in desperate need of Christian lives.

Many social leaders have emphasized the value of spirituality and love in planning utopian-type communities.[13] These societies are based on the idea that success in communal living comes more from feelings of brotherhood than on actual formal rules or practices. O'Connell called this "humanistic identification", which is an appreciation by each person that he or she is a part of a brotherhood.[14] Key parts in creating this feeling of belongingness are a consideration and a thoughtfulness for others. Thus, there is a commitment to brotherhood, obviously overlapping a main Christian theme. God's plan is to use virtuous people to save the world.

Empirical Evidence

The previous discussions have emphasized the logical arguments that religion will improve personal health and happiness, as well as lead to benefits for society. There is empirical evidence that the benefits in theory are actually found in life. Those who practice Christianity will enjoy better mental health than those who do not.[15] The summary book by Paloutzian and Park presents rather consistent conclusions that the practice of religion is related to better mental health and feelings of well-being.[16] Moreover, the scientific conclusion is that the practice of religion actually causes mental health.

The specific study of the Heritage Foundation, reported by Morphew, was previously discussed in Chapter 1.[17] That study found, for example, that those persons who engaged regularly in some form of religious practice tended to live longer, to be happier and to have higher self-esteem. Moreover, as Morphew reported:

> If you regularly attend religious worship services, your marriage will have more stability, your moral code will be stronger and you'll have fewer bouts with depression. The study also says religious people are not as likely to get killer diseases. As you can see, the benefits of regular religious practice are immense.[18]

Therefore, the results of empirical science, and the logic of religion, both support the thesis that practicing your religion will improve your quality of life.

Conclusion

None of us are securely and completely and finally in the category of committed Christian. We hang more tinsel on ourselves than we are willing to admit. Who would deny that he or she has a need to seek higher ground? We should do our best to shed the tinsel on the outside, and let the Christian light that is within us shine through in our service to others. We must do this because we can do no other. To do some other thing is to forfeit any possible reward on earth or in Heaven.

In the above paragraph, I deny once more that a person can experience a moment of total commitment to Christ—i.e., "be saved"—that can insulate him or her in some sort of sinless cocoon for the rest of his or her life. I cannot find that particular message in the Bible. But, I find many contrary messages.

How do we know that we have fulfilled God's wishes for us? The answer to that question was given to me by a friend, who is not a renowned scholar, but undoubtedly a dedicated Christian lady. She said that, during her bedtime prayer, she told the Lord that she had done her best that day to be a Christian, and, if she had not, for God to tell her so. Then, she listened for the answer with open mind and heart, trying to put aside psychological defense mechanisms of denial, rationalization and so forth. If, then, there was peace and joy in her heart, she went to sleep knowing that she had received God's answer. She had received God's greatest wages for a life on earth: peace of conscience and joy of victory.

Notes

1. Holy Bible, New International Version (Grand Rapids, MI: Zondervan Publishing House, 1973), John 3: 16.
2. Holy Bible, Matthew 5: 1-12.
3. Holy Bible, 2 Corinthians 5: 1-2.
4. E. Rae Harcum and Ellen F. Rosen, Perceived dignity as a function of perceived voluntary control of behavior. *Journal of Psychology,* 124, (1990), 495-511.
5. Holy Bible, Galatians 5, 22-23.
6. E. Rae Harcum, *Saving Our Church: Five Systemic Diseases Pose a Vital Mission for the Organized Church* (Lanham, MD: Hamilton Books, 2009).
7. W. Laurance Ventis, The relationships between religion and mental health. *Journal of Social Issues,* 5 (2) (1992), 33-48.
8. Abraham H. Maslow, Humanistic science and transcendental experiences. *Journal of Humanistic Psychology,* 5 (1965), 219-227.
9. Holy Bible, John 14: 27.
10. Holy Bible, Philippians 4: 8-9.
11. Jim Henderson and Matt Casper, *Jim and Casper go to Church: Frank Conversations About Faith, Churches, and Well-Meaning Christians* (Carol Stream, IL: Barna Books, 2007).
12. *ibid*, 167-168.
13. H. Winthrop, Humanistic psychology and intentional community. *Journal of Humanistic Psychology*, 2, (1962), 41-55.
14. W. O'Connell, Practicing Christianity and humanistic identification. *Journal of Humanistic Psychology,* 4, (1964), 118-129.
15. Ventis, The relationships between religion and mental health.
16. Raymond F. Paloutzian and Crystal L. Park, eds. *Handbook of the Psychology of Religion and Spirituality* (New York: The Guilford Press, 2005).
17. Clark Morphew, Religion must hit the streets to change U. S. attitudes. *Daily Press*, Newport News, VA, February 23, 1996, D3.
18. *ibid*.

Chapter 10

Triumphant Living

This chapter emphasizes that for successful living on this earth each person must be committed to love. A strong faith provides the necessary basis for triumphant living because love begets love. Love validates our ticket to heaven, and it also enriches our life on earth. Thus, the sharing of love must have a tremendous positive psychological effect on everyone.

In giving and receiving love, Jesus is our mentor and model. As Willard says,

> I think we finally have to say that Jesus' enduring relevance is based on his historically proven ability to speak to, to heal and empower the individual human condition. He matters because of what he brought and what he still brings to *ordinary* human beings, living their ordinary lives and coping daily with their surroundings. He promises wholeness for their lives. In sharing our weakness, he gives us strength and imparts through his companionship a life that has the quality of eternity.
>
> He comes where we are, and he brings us the life we hunger for.[1]

But, be sure that no amount of Christian love can ensure that we will not have moments of sadness and despair. The natural consequences of life are that floods and earthquakes and death will inevitably happen to destroy our joy in life. To be sure, the Christian should be sad when misfortune falls upon any of God's children.

Therefore, there can never be uninterrupted feelings of triumphant living. Moreover, the universal problem of the suffering servant to God's people is that he or she is certain to make mistakes as he or she strives to help. It seems, therefore, that we are doomed forever to feeling moments of guilt for failing to live up to the call that God has given to us.

So, because we are not perfect, some periods of guilt feelings are normal for us. Indeed, some guilt is actually a part of a normal and productive Christian life. Otherwise, we would be like the Pharisee who tried to thank God that he was not a sinner like others around him. I call that arrogant idea, which Jesus directly condemned, the "Pharisee Fallacy." Jesus not only strongly condemned the Pharisee, He actually praised the confessed sinner who pleaded for forgiveness. The praise was not for the sin, of course, but for the valid confession of it.

Defining "Triumphant"

So, if we are ordained to feel some guilt, then how is a triumphant life even possible? To begin an answer, we must examine the word "triumphant." The word means to rejoice over a victory, to be exultant, to manifest a state of joy as a result of a success. For the Christian, a victory is to resist the temptation to sin. The sin may be simple indifference to the suffering and needs of others. Or, it might be an unwillingness to help others. It is a sin of omission to withhold the help one can give when it is within one's capability to take positive action.

Therefore, a victory does not require that an action is successful in defeating the enemies of God, or in stopping the persecutors of His people. The victory is in doing one's best to accomplish the will of God. Therefore, triumphant living means to have committed oneself fully to Christian love, and so to achieve mostly victories over the temptations to sin.

The above interpretation of triumphant Christian living does not mean that the Christian can simply bask every day in the glory of past victorious events. The Christian must take on new challenges as they appear. We can hardly exult in yesterday's victory if today we are soundly defeated.

But, even in apparent defeat, we can still have final victory. We know that, if we earnestly repent of our sin, we are assured that God will forgive us. Therefore, we need never feel defeat and guilt for long, because we only have to ask to be forgiven. Thus, God through His grace grants triumphant living to those who truly believe and trust in Him, and try to do His will.

Because your defeats are erased by forgiveness if you simply repent, you can actually have an effective record of only victories. This guarantee of ultimate victories means that the Christian attitude will entail peace, optimism and happiness.

This interpretation tells us how triumphant Christian living is thus consistent with our call as Christians to be suffering servants. Never is the Christian given the promise that he or she will have a life of eternal ease and prosperity on this earth. No life is without some pain and personal trials. God does not promise that we will not die. He does not promise that we will have freedom from pain and want in this earthly life. Instead, we are promised peace of soul. We are promised a peace of the spirit that can prevail despite frequent stresses and harassments from the physical environment.

You see, a triumphant life on this earth does not mean that every moment will be a joyous celebration. The celebrations will come only after trials and periods of anguish that test our faith. Christians feel the suffering of peoples about them, and are led to helpful action by that empathy. Thus, merely to take action, to enter the fray with full Christian commitment in behalf of others, constitutes a personal victory for the Christian. Earthly defeats are merely spurs to help us achieve better actions. Thus, the suffering servant is triumphant because the suffering is temporary and trivial compared to the joys of victory over apathy and indifference.

This picture of triumphant living shows that the Christian experiences peace and happiness as the bottom line of life, the ultimate sum of living. It does not mean that the Christian does not owe debts to God and to fellow human beings.

But, it does mean that the balance sheet of life holds a very favorable credit balance of personal happiness for the person who fights the good fight and runs the course approved by the Lord.

There have been times in my life when well-meaning friends have said to me that I should just refuse to get involved in some situation where I think that wrong is being done, and therefore is causing suffering to some of God's people. In the eyes of the world, the personal rewards of victory would be too small, and the chances of defeat and humiliation would be far too great. Also, there are those who said that it was stupid of me to think even that a wrong was being committed. Therein lies a major temptation to the Christian. If you fail to identify a wrong because you simply look away from it, or you rationalize that it is not your duty or ability to identify wrongs, you can avoid the scars of a fight. But, you will not live happy, because you have not served.

Sometimes, I gained the Christian victory by doing my best, even though I may have been defeated in my attempt to solve the objective problem. Or, at least, so it may have appeared at first. Perhaps, my effort inspired a victory in the life of another, albeit unnoticed by anyone at the time.

In any case, one thing is sure: I was spared the sin and guilt of inaction, and I thus enjoyed the fruits of such triumphant living. You see, the real battle is against oneself. Does the person himself or herself struggle to do the Christian act, to right a wrong, help the helpless or demonstrate God's love in service? The true triumph, then, is winning this personal battle.

Need I add that such consistent effort to be a Godly person will also produce, as a natural consequence, many victories over evils in the world? The very effort makes the world a better place. To be sure, we will probably not win many battles if we do not get involved.

Unfortunately, there were also too many times that I failed to meet the challenge of Christian living. Perhaps, I feared personal hurt and humiliation. I thus robbed others of the chances that I might have succeeded, and myself of the additional joys of personal triumph. You see, Christian living is a no-lose choice because you are *always* a winner. There is no long-term gamble in Christian living; the result is always an ultimate favorable balance of joy and peace. That is surely a valuable message for personal mental health. In the words of James: "Blessed is the man who perseveres under trial, because when he has stood the test, he will receive the crown of life that God has promised to those who love him."[2]

I do not mean to urge a person to become a Christian because of the great personal gain from triumphant living. It does not work that way. One cannot cheat God, convince Him that one is a Christian simply to gain the rewards of worldly victory. Such thinking is blasphemy. There is no bypassing the Great Commandment to love. I am saying that the display of love—agape'—is the best policy, the greatest principle of business management, the touchstone of successful interpersonal relationships, the very essential backbone of triumphant living.

Just a World

But it is not just justice that we are serving. We should not blindly accept what psychologists and philosophers call the "just-world hypothesis," which states that good things happen to good people, and bad things happen to bad people. The belief in this hypothesis can actually be a two-edged sword: it can comfort you in your righteousness, to be sure, but it can produce anger and guilt when bad things happen to good people. Moreover, it can cause us to blame the victims.

I prefer what I call the "just-a-world hypothesis," which says that our earthly habitat is just a world, with large shares of triumph and tragedy, pleasure and pain, comfort and terror, beauty and ugliness. It surely is not Heaven. God ordained the laws by which our earth operates. And I am truly convinced that the belief in a just world is generally correct in the long run. The evils that people do will usually produce adverse consequences for them.

But, the old Hebrew idea that all calamity is a punishment by God is not true, as can be seen by anyone with open eyes and an open mind. To be sure, unless God intervenes in a specific case, the natural operation of His laws will occasionally produce innocent victims. The reason is that God loves everyone, even the sinner. He does not operate by the just-world hypothesis. Such a hypothesis is purely a human invention. Jesus said in the Sermon on the Mount:

> You have heard that it was said, 'Love your neighbor and hate your enemy.' But I tell you: love your enemies and pray for those who persecute you, that you may be sons of your Father in heaven. He causes his sun to rise on the evil and the good, and sends rain on the righteous and the unrighteous.[3]

Therefore, God loves everyone fully. I do not think that He ordinarily suspends His laws on earth in order just to save saints, or to punish sinners. Surely, God wants everyone to be healthy and happy. Undoubtedly, He originally established the laws of the universe with love for His people in mind. Therefore, His laws are best for us, although inevitably some people are hurt in the natural process. More are hurt than is necessary when people disobey the guidance from His commandments. It does not seem reasonable that God would, very often, suspend His established physical laws in order to reward some of his children on an individual basis through miracles and to punish others also through the same miracles.

It is not for us to know when or where God will decide to intervene. My personal explanation is that God is sparing in His interventions in order to keep His world orderly for us. The appearance of miracles surely confounds our scientific minds. In the same way, the laws of our legal system must be consistently enforced by police and prosecuting attorneys, or they are not truly laws. If laws were sometimes enforced, and sometimes not, they would provide no guidance for our behaviors. Similarly, God's natural laws for the universe would provide no guidance for us if He routinely suspended them when the outcome would sadden Him. In fact, physical laws that were routinely cancelled by miracles would no longer be valid principles for our guidance.

Guilt

As mentioned above, a part of God's plan is for us to be able to feel the pain of guilt. He gave us the ability to feel remorse in order to help us to stay on His path. The triumphal feeling of personal victory is not possible without the reality of guilt from losing the personal battle with sin. And such guilt is productive.

Productive Guilt

Jesus made the point that some feeling of guilt was a mark of a Christian. To some who were confident of their own righteousness and looked down on everybody else, Jesus told this parable:

> Two men went up to the temple to pray, one a Pharisee and the other a tax collector. The Pharisee stood up and prayed about himself: 'God, I thank you that I am not like other men—robbers, evildoers, adulterers—or even like this tax collector. I fast twice a week and give a tenth of all I get.'
>
> But the tax collector stood at a distance. He would not even look up to heaven, but beat his breast and said, 'God, have mercy on me, a sinner.'
>
> I tell you that this man, rather than the other, went home justified before God. For everyone who exalts himself will be humbled, and he who humbles himself will be exalted.[4]

So, guilt is normal and it can be productive. In fact, the psychiatric manual that describes the various recognized categories of disordered thinking, lists the category of anti-social personality disorder, which is an inability to feel guilt.[5] In earlier systems, persons with this disorder were called by the more familiar terms of psychopaths or sociopaths. Such persons cannot feel guilt for their anti-social behaviors, and they have no regard for the rights of others. They are characterized by deceitful behaviors and manipulations of others for personal gain.

Therefore, to feel absolutely no guilt is not normal. Actually, an ability to feel some guilt is necessary for a person to function successfully in society. Sooner or later, despite various clever tactics to hide the lack of a conscience, the functional disorder in thinking is revealed. Then, the person faces various social, and perhaps legal, sanctions that can interfere drastically with his or her success and happiness in life. Society, particularly the Christian community, holds the person accountable for losing his or her internal personal battle.

And it is here that we get back to the need for spiritual health. To feel guilt, one must first have some personal standards or criteria for moral or ethical behaviors, whether these standards come from religious or some other moral or ethical system.

Debilitating Guilt

The presence of guilt can also have a debilitating side, of course, especially when it is excessive with respect to the severity of the offense. To be sure, God does not want us to be so burdened with guilt that we are stuck along the way, mired down, unable to help either ourselves or others. In fact, such a freezing of action also actually entails psychological pathology. The psychiatric manual of thinking disorders does not include a specific single category that is the exact opposite of the antisocial personality disorder. The opposite category would include a person who was excessively loaded with feelings of guilt. Actually, there are several categories in the diagnostic system that reflect an excessive preoccupation or over-burdening with perceived guilt. One example is the mood disorder of depression, in which the person is chronically depressed beyond appropriate reason. The diagnosis of this category recognizes that there are some unfortunate situations, such as loss of a loved one, loss of job, major financial setback and so forth, which would cause any reasonable person to become depressed for an appropriate period of time. Such is *not* clinical depression. In fact, under such circumstances of severe loss or disappointment, we would suspect pathology if the person were not depressed for a reasonable period of time. Although the sorrow may well continue, the depression will disappear for the Christian, because of the blessed assurance of God's love and peace.

Another category of disordered thinking includes several anxiety disorders, in which the person has worries and fears that again are not reasonable under the circumstances. A major part of such diagnoses is that the person is impaired in his or her ability to function adequately within his or her society.

As we all know, guilt is stressful. It can arouse and it can distract us from the work at hand. The arousal can actually benefit our work if it is not too severe because it can spur us on to greater effort and productive activity. Yet, if the stress is too great, the level of arousal exceeds the level that is most efficient for the job. Then, the excessive guilt is harmful to effective performance, because it does not lend itself to the discriminations that are necessary for selecting the best course of action from among many possible alternatives. Thus, the ability to solve problems is impaired.

Such impairment of functioning in life is contrary, I think, to the will of God. He desires all of His children to be happy and productive. His plan and desire is for each person to be effective enough to help others who are not yet so effective. Therefore, it is not reasonable for a person to sabotage his or her effective functioning in the world in some sort of ill-advised, self-injurious attempt to appease God.

Managing Guilt

The natural conclusion from the above paragraphs is that psychologically normal functioning in our society requires some degree of an ability to feel guilt, but not too much. Then, we ask: how much? The answer to that question depends upon what level of guilt will produce the most productive behaviors for that individual person. I believe that the truly productive response is the Christian response. That is, Christian behavior is always best for the long-term interests of the individual, as well as for the society. God wants us to feel guilty when we have not followed His teaching to love Him and to love our fellow human beings as ourselves. When we sin and repent, God forgives us, and helps us to forgive ourselves. And this process is psychologically healthful.

If a person is too stressed to function effectively, the problem is to find ways to reduce the stress. There are three general ways, which are not mutually exclusive: (1) Cease the behaviors that are producing the guilt; (2) Change the evaluation of the behaviors such that they produce less guilt; and (3) Accept that God forgives when we earnestly repent.

If the behaviors are truly unacceptable ethically, then the person must simply muster his or her personal spiritual power (courage) to win the personal battle. This can be achieved through prayer, study, counseling, support of friends and whatever else that might work for the individual person.

If the person is evaluating a situation in a way that causes him or her to feel unnecessary guilt or pain, then a cognitive re-evaluation of the situation is appropriate. So, good advice for the sufferer is to try to look at the situation objectively in order to assess the reality. You may ask: are my negative feelings really appropriate?

The issue of when and how one should try to change the attitudes and feelings of a friend is very delicate. On the one hand, as a friend, you are naturally inclined to want to help your neighbor who is needlessly distressed by a situation in life. You desperately want to talk him or her out of the distressing interpretation of a condition in life. This is what friends do.

On the other hand, the advice about attitude is the most sensitive in terms of the dangers in attempting to practice psychotherapy. The loving friend can reasonably go so far as to raise the possibility that a different interpretation of the facts is possible. The friend may express his or her different interpretation of the facts. For example, all mistakes are not sins that deserve feelings of guilt. But, the advice must not go into a deeper analysis of the friend's habitual mode of thinking. The helping friend must stick to objective reality as most people would view reality.

Obviously, this is a most difficult task, requiring the most careful discrimination. The danger is in arousing even more disturbing thoughts in the troubled friend, thoughts that the usual friend is not prepared to handle. Therefore, the caring friend is advised to stay on the safe side of any question about proper personal attitudes and feelings. Be assured that you can do no harm by being genuine, expressing empathy and providing unconditional love as a Christian neighbor.

Inappropriate interpretation of life situations very often requires professional help. For example, questions about why someone is making an inappropriate interpretation surely requires professional help. If a non-professional friend foolishly tries to dig into such issues, he or she may awaken dormant problems of adjustment that could potentially provide serious personal problems. To take an extreme case, as a student, I once remarked to a psychiatric patient that she seemed to be doing quite well in her current situation. That seemingly innocent remark set her off into a paranoid episode of personal persecution, which I, as a beginning student, was not equipped to handle.

Professional psychotherapists are trained to change inappropriate cognitions in a safe manner. Many of them find the use of religious thought helpful in such therapy. As Helmeke and Ford say,

> We also urge readers to be sensitive as they apply these various exercises to clients of different backgrounds. We reiterate the concern we raised in the introduction to the first book: that therapists need to exercise care when integrating spirituality in therapy so they do not impose their religious beliefs and values onto their clients. . . We endorse these concerns and urge readers, prior to even attempts to use any of the interventions described, to first examine themselves in the ways described in many of the chapters, and then to assess their clients' openness and readiness to incorporate spirituality in therapy.[6]

It should be kept in mind that Helmeke and Ford were writing for professional therapists, not for loving friends.

Finally, the sinner must constantly remember that God understands and forgives. He does not want us to lapse into unproductive guilt when we have done our best to follow His commandment. But, He does want us to feel productive guilt when we fail to feed His sheep, to connect with one another in His world, to love one another.

Such productive guilt does not cause us to become moody and depressed, but energizes us to Christ-like action. So, we tell everything to God in prayer, ask for forgiveness and accept the forgiveness when it is given. Thus, true repentance produces a clean slate.

Positive Thinking

The term, "positive thinking," was made popular by Norman Vincent Peale.[7] Peale's message was simply that self confidence and a belief that one can conquer certain obstacles to successful and happy living will actually help the person to overcome those obstacles. Peale called the process simply "applied Christianity."

I cannot add much to Peale's appeal, except anecdotal support from my own experience. Specifically, there have been times in my life when some event occurred that I considered at the time to be totally disastrous to my happiness and to my future. For example, there were numerous times in my youth when I thought that a particular member of the opposite gender was absolutely indispensable to my future happiness. All but one of these young ladies actually turned out not to be necessary. In fact, the mistakes and rejections over the years provided me with the opportunity to evaluate what I had to offer a potential mate. Thus, these painful learning experiences helped me grow so that I was better prepared later for the successful relationship that I now enjoy, and have enjoyed for over 57 years. A major part of my success was to have selected a mate who had the tools and heart to make the marriage work. Psychologically, it may be as valuable to learn what does not work in interpersonal relationships as it is to find out what produces a success.

The same conclusion can be reached with respect to apparent career setbacks. For example, after graduate school in Michigan, I was hoping for an opportunity to work in Virginia, where I grew up and where my parents and inlaws lived. Therefore, I was delighted to obtain an interview for a job in Virginia, one that was a good match for my qualifications. But, I was not hired. Naturally, I was totally dejected, because I was sure that such a good opportunity would never come again. Then, unbelievably, a week later a call came from the chairman of the psychology department at The College of William and Mary, my alma mater in Virginia, informing me that a position in my area of expertise had unexpectedly come open. And I got the job! Needless to say, if I had taken the other job the week before, I would not have been free to accept the William and Mary job, which I naturally preferred. What a blessing it was to be able to move to a position that was within 30 miles of my wife's ancestral home.

Such stories convince me that we cannot always tell whether a bit of news is good or bad for us until we have acquired some time perspective for evaluating it. Until you find out otherwise, I recommend the power of positive thinking.

I certainly do not propose to be positive in thinking when such thinking is unrealistic. One must identify and make concessions to the realities of life. I do think, however, that most of the time the positive approach is the realistic one. Moreover, the positive attitude can actually make good things happen, as Peale assured us.

Mental Health and Well-being

Numerous recent publications have been devoted to the topic of religious influences on personal and societal well-being.[8] Well-being has been defined to include such things as ability to cope with problems of living, mental health and physical health. The influence of religion on mental health could be either beneficial or harmful to society, depending upon many factors. This conclusion is consistent with the tenor of the book edited by Schumaker on the relationships between religion and mental health.[9] In fact, Schumaker considers the topic so complex that he refused even to make a general conclusion other than that "religion" contains the potential to produce either positive or negative effects on mental health.

Ventis discussed the psychological research on the empirical relationships between religion and mental health.[10] Consistent with Schumaker's conclusion, mentioned above, surprisingly the relationship is not always a positive one, because the nature of the relationship depends upon, first, how one defines mental health, and, second, how one defines religion.

The definition of what I call good religion approaches religion as a personal commitment to a set of convictions for letting God control one's life. This is surely the Christian approach, involving love and service to others. The definition of what I call bad religion approaches religion as merely a means for gaining selfish goals, such as emotional and social support or social status, without reference to God's will.

This difference in types of religion means, for example, that regular attendance at church is not necessarily related to better mental health. The nature of the church and the nature of the worship and faith are the things that matter for mental health.

Mental health is also exceedingly complex to define. In fact, Ventis lists seven factors to be included in the conception of mental health.[11] These factors include everything from the simple absence of mental disorders, to such characteristics as appropriate social behavior, freedom from worry and guilt, a sense of personal control and competence, self-acceptance and self-actualization, maintenance of unifying principles in one's life and open-mindedness and flexibility of attitudes.

Ventis concluded that the empirical evidence on the positive relationship between mental health and religion favors what I have called good religion. For example, 48 out of 49 psychological studies revealed a negative (inverse) relationship between practicing *bad* religion and a measure of mental health. In sharp contrast, 49 of 63 research studies revealed a positive relationship between *good* religion and mental health.

These relationships are the Paradox of Christian Living in action! I conclude that those who try to use religion to achieve extrinsic personal goals are actually less likely to achieve those personal goals. In sharp contrast, those persons who seek to live according to personal convictions of right and wrong are actually more likely to achieve those same personal goals. These data present a most powerful convergence of Biblical and scientific truths.

The same general conclusions apply to religion as a community resource. For example, Maton and Wells conclude that religion tends to be an important resource outreach to families and children for the prevention of problems in the community, for the healing of existing problems and for the empowerment of certain social groups that tend to suffer discrimination from society.[12]

To be sure, some harmful practices can be conducted in the name of religion. For example, the power of religion can be perverted by bureaucrats to weaken certain groups and to compete for material resources in the secular community. Such negative effects are admittedly not due to religion, but to individuals who lose sight of sound religious teachings in their attempt to practice their form of religion in the community.

Accepting Help

Although stress reduction is usually a do-it-yourself project, nevertheless often professional help is needed. Sometimes the stress is like quicksand, in which the victim cannot save himself or herself because there is no solid support to grasp in order to pull oneself out. In such a case, outside help is needed. Such help may be in the form of a professional who is specifically trained in psychology or religion, or both, or it may even be a wise and caring friend.

Do not refuse help when you need it. It makes as much sense to refuse needed help of a psychological sort as it would be to refuse to grab a hand or a lifeline if you were stuck in quicksand.

Christian Atmosphere

We often hear a person described as pleasant to be around, because he or she creates a desired atmosphere, an ambient aura of good feeling that other people want to experience. This characteristic includes such attributes as self-confidence, good disposition, a good sense of humor, a ready smile, an absence of complaining, a tendency to give nice compliments, a willingness to connect in a positive way with other people and so forth. It does not mean that the person is wildly optimistic, or unrealistic, but just generally positive in attitudes about life.

Such people tend to be liked, and thus their presence sought by other people. Therefore, they are eminently successful in their interpersonal relations. The principle here is what psychologists call the "law of effect," which says that responses leading to a satisfying internal state of affairs will tend to be repeated. Therefore, if being around you makes a person feel good, he or she will tend to take some action to be around you. Accordingly, if you wish to be popular, then send out a good feeling tone—one that flows from a Christian life. Try to connect in a positive way. Personal popularity can be as simple as that.

But, remember, if your goal is just to be popular, rather than to love, your plan will not work. Other people will discover that you are not genuine. This again is the Paradox of Christian Living.

Therefore, one of the major secrets of triumphant living is to see to it that you emanate good feelings in all of your connections with other people. And the point is this: I can think of no better way to ensure that you will emanate a good atmosphere than to attempt to apply your Christianity in your everyday living. If you love yourself and others as God loves you and them, you will have the right approach for creating a good atmosphere of love among everyone around you. And you will notice that those around you will return in kind, to add to your personal happiness.

This point has been verified by formal psychological research.[13] The purpose of a study by Calvin was to show that college-student behavior could be established by having the students' peers compliment them for performing a particular behavior. The chosen behavior was the wearing of a given color of clothing. It was presumed that there would be no moral issue in changing such trivial behavior.

The predicted result was indeed obtained, but another important effect was also incidentally discovered. The students who were given the job of making the compliments found that their personal popularity also clearly improved. By creating good feelings in their classmates from giving the rewards, they themselves had become associated with those good feelings in the minds of their classmates. This positive connection occurred even though the experimenters did not set out to make it happen. This was indeed an unexpected, but pleasant, side effect of administering rewards.

One of my own experiences illustrates this same point. I was quite surprised a few years ago to receive a card from a recent graduate of our master's degree program at William and Mary because, being retired, I had not been her teacher. Although I spent a substantial amount of time in the psychology building, I really did not know her well. She thanked me for merely greeting her pleasantly and smiling when I passed her in the hallways of the psychology department during her time in graduate school. She said that there were times in her life as a graduate student when her spirits were low, and my friendly greetings gave her a little helpful lift in spirits. Similarly, her greeting and friendly smile had always been a welcome addition to my day.

I had not singled her out to be a special connection. I was indeed unaware of any therapeutic value of my behaviors. I was not attempting to do psychotherapy or promote mental health. But, surely, the effect was there. All of us have days in which friendly greetings and smiles are badly needed. Give one, and get one in return. That is triumphant living at absolutely no personal cost. And, indeed the reward is abundant.

The reward incidentally promotes mental health. Even without the deliberate intention of providing psychological benefit to another, that is exactly what it does. The reward makes one feel good, strong and capable. It gives one the confidence to give service and to accept service from others. It induces one to model his or her behavior after the person giving the love.

Discussion

Truly, we receive all good things through God's grace. The action that is required of us is that we open ourselves to the reception. Therefore, the action of opening oneself to receive God's blessings is not the same as a selfish search for those blessings. There must be a graceful acceptance of gifts that one has desired, but not worked for directly. This, as I have said, is the Paradox of Christian Living.

This chapter thus completes the circle. It contends that the person who loves

God, and has developed the ability to love others as well as himself or herself, will enjoy improved circumstances in life. This improvement is general, including earthly treasures, such as business success, social standing, and physical and mental wellness. But, it must be remembered, such a state of personal happiness on earth does not represent rewards for good behavior in the psychological sense of extrinsic rewards. Rather, it is merely a natural direct consequence of the love and service to others.

It is perhaps ironic that at the end of this book, I conclude with the comments made by Matt Casper, an avowed atheist who completed a book with Pastor Jim Henderson, which summarized their dialogues after jointly attending various Christian services across the country.[14] Casper's meaningful summary was as follows:

> Jim asked me what I'd say to Christians everywhere if I could, and I think it's quite simple. There are two rules we must all abide by to live healthy, happy lives with each other and with everyone on the planet:
>
> 1. Be open-minded. Learning is the best thing that can happen to any one.
> 2. Do unto others as you would have them do unto you.
>
> And, though I've never met the man, I think Jesus would agree.[15]

Thus, the best policy for peace and joy on earth is to follow the guidance of love. The fruits of righteousness, which stem from love, are described in Proverbs:

> My son, if you accept my words and store up my commands within you,
> turning your ear to wisdom and applying your heart to understanding,
> and if you call out for insight and cry loud for understanding,
> and if you look for it as for silver and search for it as for hidden treasure,
> then you will understand the fear of the LORD and find the knowledge of God.
> For the LORD gives wisdom, and from his mouth come knowledge and understanding.
> He holds victory in store for the upright, he is a shield to those whose walk is blameless,
> For he guards the course of the just and protects the way of his faithful ones.
> Then you will understand what is right and just and fair—every good path.
> For wisdom will enter your heart, and knowledge will be plea-

sant to your soul.
Discretion will protect you, and understanding will guard you.[16]

As I said, to serve in love for others is a no-lose situation. And, as Proverbs says, the victory (intrinsic reward) that results from it is very sweet. And, in this way, your love for others truly provides the fruits of mental health for yourself and for others.

Notes

1. Dallas Willard, *The Divine Conspiracy: Rediscovering our Hidden Life in God* (New York: Harper San Francisco, 1998), 13.
2. Holy Bible, New International Version, (Grand Rapids, MI: Zondervan Publishing House, 1973), James 1: 12.
3. Holy Bible, Matthew 5: 43-45.
4. Holy Bible, Luke 18: 9-14.
5. American Psychiatric Association, *Diagnostic and Statistical Manual DSM-IV* (4th ed.) (Washington, DC: American Psychiatric Association, 1994).
6. K. B. Helmeke and S. C. Ford, eds. *The Therapists' Notebook for Integrating Spirituality in Counseling* (Binghamton, NY: The Haworth Press, 2006), xxvii.
7. Norman V. Peale, *The Power of Positive Thinking* (New York: Fawcett Crest, 1956).
8. For example, *Handbook of the Psychology of Religion and Spirituality,* eds. Raymond F. Paloutzian and Crystal Park (New York: The Guilford Press, 2005).
9. J. F. Schumacher, ed. *Religion and Mental Health* (New York: Oxford University Press, 1992).
10. W. Laurance Ventis, The relationships between religion and mental health, *Journal of Social Issues. 5* (2), 1992, 33-48.
11. *ibid.*
12. K. I. Maton and E. A. Wells, Religion as a community resource for well-being: prevention, healing and empowerment pathways. *Journal of Social Issues, 51* (2), 1995, 177-193.
13. A. D. Calvin, Social reinforcement. *The Journal of Social Psychology,* 56, 1962, 15-18.
14. Jim Henderson and Matt Casper, *Jim and Casper go to Church: Frank Conversation about Faith, Churches, and Well-Meaning Christians* (Carol Stream, IL: Barna Books, 2007).
15. *ibid*, 154.
16. Holy Bible, Proverbs 2: 1-11.

PART V. FINAL WORDS

Final Words

As parting words, I wish to leave the reader with four particular ideas:
(1) Christian living necessarily begins with love as the driving motivation. Love provides the power of virtue. If your heart is not in the right place, your behavior will not get you to the right place, and you will not be able to help anyone.
(2) You must develop and follow your own conscience, guided by your love. No human being on earth can give you rules for good behavior, which, if followed exactly, will achieve your dream of Christian living.
(3) Do not become discouraged if your conscience tells you that you often fail. Know that God is a forgiving God. Though He calls upon you to be perfect, He knows that you cannot be blameless. He asks you to try. The very act of trying becomes triumphant Christian living.
(4) Finally, with the assurance of God's love, grace and forgiveness, comes a feeling of personal security. The stress of life disappears when we have the confidence to know that we can handle it because God is for us. As Paul said to the Romans, "If God is for us, who can be against us?"[1] This gift of peace is wonderfully expressed at many places in the Psalms. I will quote just one of them.

> I will praise the Lord, who counsels me; even at night my heart instructs me.
> I have set the Lord before me. Because he is at my right hand, I will not be shaken.
> Therefore, my heart is glad and my tongue rejoices; my body also will rest secure.
> Because you will not abandon me to the grave, nor will you let your Holy One decay.
> You have made known to me the path of life; you will fill me with joy in your presence, with eternal pleasures at your right hand.[2]

Notes

1. Holy Bible, New International Version (Grand Rapids, MI: Zondervan Publishing House, 1973), Romans 8:31.
2. Holy Bible, Psalm 16, 7-11.

Bibliography

American Psychiatric Association. *Diagnostic and Statistical Manual*. DSM-IV (4th ed.). Washington, DC: American Psychiatric Association, 1994.

Beck, Joan. "The frustrating job of ending a culture of violence." *Daily Press* September 10, 1994, A8.

Blackaby, Henry T., and King, C. V. *Experiencing God*. Nashville, TN: Broadman & Holman Publishers, 1994.

Booth, W. "Forgiveness may not lead to real reconciliation." *Daily Press*, September 27, 1997, D7.

Calvin, A. D. "Social reinforcement." *The Journal of Social Psychology, 56*, (1962): 15-19.

Carneal, Russell M. "Ethics of a jurist," in *Biblical Guidance and Human Choices*, edited by E. R. Harcum, 233-239. Willliamsburg, VA: Cape Books (1999).

Clay, Rebecca A. "Psychologists' faith in religion begins to grow." *A.P.A. Monitor, 27 (8), (1),* 1996a: 48.

——"Religion and psychology share ideals and beliefs." *A.P.A. Monitor, 27 (8)*, 1996b: 47.

Enroth, Ronald M. *Churches That Abuse*. Grand Rapids, MI: Zondervan Publishing House, 1992.

Freud, Sigmund. *An Outline of Psychoanalysis*. J. Strachey, trans., New York: Norton, 1949.

Glasser, William. *Reality Therapy*. New York: Harper & Row, 1965.

Hall, M. H. "An interview with 'Mr. Humanist.'" Rollo May. *Psychology Today*, 1, (1967): 24-29; 72-73.

Harcum, E. Rae. *Exploration and learning in a three-dimensional maze by rats with restricted experience in one dimension*. PhD. dissertation, University of Michigan Microfilms, Publ. No. 12581, 1955.

——*Psychology for Daily Living*. Chicago: Nelson-Hall, 1979.

——"Defensive reactance of psychologists to a metaphysical foundation for integrating different psychologies." *The Journal of Psychology, 122* (1988), 217-235.

——"The relative utility of complementary disparate views on voluntarism and determinism." *The Journal of Psychology*, *125*, (1988): 217-235.

——"Behavioral paradigm for a psychological resolution of the free will issue." *The Journal of Mind and Behavior*, 12, (1991), 93-114.

——*A psychology of freedom and dignity*. Westport, CT: Praeger, 1994.

——"Implications of the contradictions in behaviorism for a scientifically based public policy," in *The Integration of Psychological Principles in Policy Development*, edited by C. E. Stout, 173-183. Westport, CT: Praeger, 1995.

——*Biblical Guidance and Human Choices*, edited by E. Rae Harcum, Williamsburg, VA: Cape Books, 1999.

——*The Incidental Psychotherapy in Christian Connection.* (unpublished manuscript.)

——*Saving Our Church: Five Systemic Disease Pose a Vital Mission for the Organized Church.* Lanham, MD: Hamilton Books, 2009.

——Burijon, B. N., and Watson, N. "Client responsibility in the practitioners' operational definition of behavior therapy." *Journal of Human Behavior and Learning, 5,* (1988): 12-16.

——and Rosen, E. F. "Perceived dignity as a function of perceived voluntary control of behaviors." *Journal of Psychology, 124,* (1990): 495-511.

——and Rosen, E. F., Pilkington, C. J., and Petty, L. C. "An external validation of laboratory evidence for earned dignity." *Journal of Applied Social Psychology, 25,* (1995): 1204-1213.

Hart, Thomas. *Hidden Spring: The Spiritual Dimension of Therapy* (2nd ed.). Minneapolis: Fortress Press, 2002.

Hartz, Gary W. *Spirituality and Mental Health: Clinical Applications.* Binghamton, NY: The Haworth Press, 2009.

Hebb, Donald O. *The Organization of Behavior.* New York: Wiley, 1949.

Helmeke, K. B. and Ford. S. C., editors of *The Therapists' Notebook for Integrating Spirituality in Counseling.* Binghamton, NY: The Haworth Press, 2006.

Henderson, Jim, and Casper, Matt. *Jim and Casper go to Church: Frank Conversation about Faith, Churches, and Well-Meaning Christians.* Carol Stream, IL: Barna Books, 2007.

Holy Bible, New International Version. Grand Rapids, MI: Zondervan Publishing House, 1973.

Kahle, P. and Robbins, J.M. *The Power of Spirituality in Therapy: Integrating Spiritual and Religious Beliefs in Mental Health Practice.* Binghamton, NY: The Haworth Press, 2004.

Kohlberg, Lawrence. "Revisions in the theory and practice of moral development," in *New Directions for Child Development*, edited by W. Damon. San Francisco: Jossey-Bass, 1978.

——Essays on moral development: Vol. 1. *The Philosophy of Moral Development.* San Francisco: Harper & Row, 1981.

Maclean, P. D., "The imitative-creative interplay of our three mentalities," in *Astride the Two Cultures*, edited by H. Harris, 187-213. London: Hutchinson, 1979.

Mahoney, Annette, and Tarakeshwar, Nalina. "Religious role in marriage and parenting in daily life and during family crises," in *Handbook of the Psychology of Religion and Spirituality*, edited by Raymond F. Paloutzian & Crystal L. Park, 177-195. New York: The Guilford Press, 2005.

Mahoney, Michael J. "Psychology and Human Change Processes, in *Cognition and Psychotherapy*, edited by M. J. Mahoney & A. Freeman, 3-48. New York: Plenum Press, 1985.

Marty, M. E., Foreword, in *Religion and American Public Life*, edited by R. W. Lovin, 1-4. New York: Paulist Press, 1986.

Maslow, Abraham H. "Humanistic Science and Transcendental Experiences." *Journal of Humanistic Psychology, 5*, (1965): 219-227.

Maton, K. I., and Wells, E. A. "Religion as a community resource for well-being: prevention, healing and empowerment pathways." *Journal of Social Issues, 51 (2)*, (1995): 177-193.

May, Rollo, in M. H. Hill, "An Interview with 'Mr. Humanist,'" Rollo May, *Psychology Today, 1*, (1967), 24-25, 72-73.

McCullough, Michael E., Bono, Giacomo, and Root, Lindsey M. "Religion and forgiveness," in *Handbook of the Psychology of Religion and Spirituality*, edited by Raymond F. Paloutzian and Crystal Park, 394-411. New York: The Guilford Press, 2005.

Miller, G. *Incorporating Spirituality into Counseling and Psychotherapy*. New York: Wiley, 2003.

Miller, George A. "Psychology as a means of monitoring human welfare." *American Psychologist, 46*, (1969) 1063-1075.

Miller, Lisa, and Kelley, Brian S. "Relationships of religiosity and spirituality with mental health and psychotherapy," in *Handbook of the Psychology of Religion and Spirituality*, edited by Raymond F. Paloutzian and Crystal L. Park, 460-478. New York: The Guilford Press, 2005.

Morphew, Clark. "Religions must hit the streets to change U. S. attitudes." *Daily Press*, Newport News, VA, February 23, 1996, D3.

O'Connell, W. "Practicing Christianity and humanistic identification." *Journal of Humanistic Psychology, 4*, (1964): 118-129.

Oman, Doug, and Thoresen, Carl E. "Do religion and spirituality influence health?," in *Handbook of the Psychology of Religion and Spirituality*, edited by Raymond F. Paloutzian and Crystal L. Park, 435-359. New York: The Guilford Press, 2005.

Paloutzian, Raymond F. and Park, Crystal L., editors of *Handbook of the Psychology of Religion and Spirituality*. New York: The Guilford Press, 2005.

Peale, N. V. *The Power of Positive Thinking*. New York: Fawcett Crest, 1956.

Peters, R. S. *Psychology and Ethical Development*. London: Geo. Allen and Union, Ltd., 1974.

Piaget, Jean. *The Child's Conception of the World*. New York: Harcourt, Brace, 1929.

Raspberry, William. "Make communities safe from and for children." *Daily Press*, August 19, 1994, A12.

Rogers, Carl R. "A theory of therapy, personality, and interpersonal relationships, as developed in the client-centered framework," in *Psychology: A Study of a Science, Vol. 3*, edited by S. Koch, 184-256. New York: McGraw-Hill, 1959.

Safranske, Edward P. "The psychology of religion in clinical and counseling psychology," in *Handbook of the Psychology of Religion and Spirituality*, edited by Raymond F. Paloutzian and Crystal L. Park, 496-514. New York:

The Guilford Press, 2005.

Schumaker, J. F., editor of *Religion and Mental Health*. New York: Oxford University Press, 1992.

Seligman, M. E. P. "Learned helplessness." *Depression: Concepts, Controversies and Some New Facts*, edited by G. J. Levitt, B. Rubin and J. Brooks. Hillsdale, NJ: Erlbaum, 1983.

Silvis, M. "Ethics in the church," in *Biblical Guidance and Human Choices*, edited by E. Rae Harcum, 27-33. Williamsburg, VA: Cape Books, 1999.

Skinner, B. F. *Science and Human Behavior*. New York: Macmillan, 1953.

Snow, Tony. "Ventura lost out with God." *Daily Press*, Newport News, VA, October 11, 1999, A15.

Sperry, L. *Spirituality in Clinical Practice: Incorporating the Spiritual Dimension in Psychotherapy and Counseling.*" New York: Brunner-Routledge, 2001.

Sullivan, Timothy J. "Wren building stands as a symbol of college's vitality." *William and Mary News, 25 (2)*, September 1, 1995, 4-5.

Ventis, W. Laurance. "The relationships between religion and mental health." *Journal of Social Issues, 5 (2)*, (1992): 33-48.

Watson, John B. "Psychology as the Behaviorist views it." *Psychological Review, 20,* (1913): 158-177.

Willard, Dallas. *The Divine Conspiracy: Rediscovering our Hidden Life in God.* New York: Harper San Francisco, 1998.

Winthrop, H. "Humanistic psychology and intentional community." *Journal of Humanistic Psychology*, (Spring, 1962): 41-55.

About the Author

E. Rae Harcum, PhD., is a professional psychologist, and a long-time member of a Protestant religious denomination. He taught psychology at the college level for many years. He has authored many journal articles in psychology, and several books on psychology and religion.